THE CASTOR OIL BIBLE

CHERYL DI FIORE

Remember to

GET YOUR FREE BONUSES!

This book comes with valuable bonuses that perfectly complement its content, offering you additional information and practical tips for even better health and beauty results.

**Scan the QR code
on the final page of this book to download them!**

TABLE OF CONTENTS

CHAPTER 7
CASTOR OIL PACKS

CHAPTER 8
CASTOR OIL RECIPES

PURPOSE AND SCOPE OF THIS BOOK

Whether you're a **holistic health enthusiast** seeking reliable, science-backed information, a **cost-conscious** consumer looking for affordable DIY solutions, or someone **wary of the chemicals** in commercial products, this book has something perfect for you.

Skeptical? You'll be amazed to learn that the chemical properties of castor oil and its interactions with cells and organs are far more than just "woo-woo" or old folklore. Your second reaction after amazement? You'll be excited to share this newfound knowledge with your family and friends, confident that you won't be taken for a fool.

Imagine healing your body and mind while comfortably resting at home or even while sleeping, or keeping up with your busy day just by wearing a cotton flannel secured under your clothing. That's why thousands of people are already devoted to castor oil and prefer it over drugs, supplements, or pharmaceuticals. And the best news is, you can too.

This book will reveal why castor oil has its effects, helping you distinguish between mere rumors and popular trends versus what's actually true with substantial evidence. Recognizing that many people have busy lives and aren't scientists, this book offers easy-to-follow explanations on every noteworthy aspect of castor oil's actions. You'll learn how castor oil can address your most common health, beauty, and wellness concerns, as well as your mental and emotional wellbeing, providing relief from stress and promoting relaxation. Some images, charts, and tables will assist in your discovery, alongside step-by-step guides to implementing routines and recipes, making this book accessible to everyone. You'll be able to incorporate these practices into your daily routine without wasting time or money.

This journey will also help you gain a deep awareness of your body as a wonderfully interconnected system. You'll learn about the key functions of your organs and how they interact in delicate balance. By understanding these mechanisms, you'll be able to stimulate your system in the best possible way to alleviate unwanted symptoms and contribute to lasting health.

INTRODUCTION

The Role of Natural Remedies

Overview

The resurgence of natural remedies in today's health and wellness conversations shows a growing appreciation for holistic approaches to well-being. This shift is based on several key factors that highlight the unique benefits of natural remedies over conventional synthetic products.

Natural remedies take a holistic approach to health, focusing not just on relieving symptoms but also on improving overall well-being. This approach considers physical, mental, emotional, and spiritual health, aiming to balance and harmonize these aspects. Unlike synthetic drugs that often target specific symptoms, natural remedies support the body's natural healing processes, fostering long-term wellness.

Many natural remedies have been used for centuries in various cultures, with their effectiveness documented in traditional medicine systems like TCM (Traditional Chinese Medicine), Ayurveda, and Indigenous medicine. The long history and widespread use of these remedies show their effectiveness and safety. This historical knowledge guides modern applications and innovations.

Benefits and Advantages over Synthetic Products

Natural remedies have significant advantages, primarily due to their lower risk of side effects compared to synthetic drugs. Synthetic drugs often come with adverse effects due to their potent active ingredients and chemical compositions. In contrast, natural remedies, derived from whole plants or natural sources, work more gently on the body, reducing the likelihood of harmful side effects. This is specifically beneficial for people with chronic conditions that require long-term treatment.

Additionally, the production of natural remedies generally has a lower environmental impact compared to synthetic pharmaceuticals. Sustainable cultivation and harvesting of medicinal plants can support biodiversity and reduce chemical pollution, aligning with increasing consumer awareness and concern for environmental conservation.

Natural remedies also offer a more personalized healthcare approach. Practitioners take the time to understand an individual's unique health profile, leading to more effective and tailored health solutions. This personalized care encourages active engagement with one's health, fostering a deeper understanding and more informed health choices.

CHAPTER 1
HISTORICAL AND MODERN USES

A Historical Perspective

Castor oil boasts a long history spanning thousands of years.

Historical records, including ancient medical texts, papyri, and manuscripts, provide detailed accounts of castor oil's applications. These documents highlight the oil's enduring value across different cultures and time periods. The consistent use of castor oil throughout history underscores its effectiveness and the deep-rooted human connection to natural remedies.

Usage in Ancient Egypt

Ancient Egypt is perhaps one of the most documented civilizations regarding the use of castor oil. The Egyptians valued castor oil for its medicinal, cosmetic, and industrial applications.

Ancient Egyptian texts, such as the Ebers Papyrus (circa 1550 BCE), detail the use of castor oil as a laxative and for treating various ailments, including eye irritations and skin conditions. The oil was also used in embalming practices and applied to wounds to promote healing. Cleopatra is said to have used castor oil as her preferred beauty treatment to enhance the whiteness of her eyes.

Egyptian women used castor oil as a beauty treatment. It was applied to the skin to maintain a youthful appearance and to the hair to enhance shine and strength. Castor oil's moisturizing properties helped protect the skin and hair from the harsh desert climate.

The ancient Egyptians also utilized castor oil as a fuel for lamps. Its ability to burn cleanly and brightly made it an ideal choice for lighting temples, homes, and tombs.

Usage in Ancient India

In ancient India, castor oil was an integral part of Ayurvedic medicine, a traditional system of healing that dates back over 3,000 years.

Ayurvedic texts such as the Charaka Samhita and Sushruta Samhita describe the use of castor oil for a variety of health issues. It was used as a purgative to cleanse the digestive system, treat joint pain and arthritis, and alleviate skin disorders.

Castor oil also played a role in various spiritual and purification rituals in ancient India. It was used in oil lamps during religious ceremonies to invoke divine blessings and create a serene atmosphere. The oil's purity and ability to sustain a long-lasting flame made it a symbol of light and knowledge in Hindu rituals.

Usage in Other Cultures

In ancient China, castor oil was used for its medicinal properties, much like in Egypt and India. Traditional Chinese medicine utilized the oil to treat ailments such as constipation, skin infections, and respiratory issues. Historical texts and pharmacopoeias from the period document its widespread use.

The ancient Greeks and Romans also recognized the benefits of castor oil. Hippocrates and Galen, two foundational figures in the history of medicine, explored the therapeutic benefits of castor oil for improving eye, skin, and oral health. The oil was used to treat wounds, skin conditions, and digestive disorders. Greek and Roman physicians often prescribed castor oil as part of their therapeutic regimens.

Various African cultures used castor oil for medicinal and cosmetic purposes. It was applied to wounds, used as a massage oil to relieve muscle pain, and employed in hair care routines to promote growth and prevent dryness. The oil's versatility made it a staple in traditional African medicine cabinets.

Industrial Uses of Castor Oil

Role in Manufacturing and Industry

Castor oil has a significant role in various industrial applications.

One of the primary industrial uses of castor oil is in the production of lubricants and hydraulic fluids. Its high lubricity and ability to maintain viscosity at both high and low temperatures make it an ideal candidate for these applications. Castor oil-based lubricants are preferred in high-performance engines, aircraft, and racing cars where consistent performance under extreme conditions is critical.

It is also a vital raw material in the production of various plastics and polymers. It serves as a monomer in the synthesis of polyurethanes, which are used to manufacture flexible foams, elastomers, and coatings. These materials are essential in automotive interiors, furniture, and footwear industries.

The paint and coating industry extensively utilizes castor oil for its ability to dry quickly and form a durable, glossy finish. It is a key ingredient in alkyd resins, which are used to produce high-quality paints and coatings. These products are widely applied in automotive, marine, and architectural applications.

In the cosmetics industry, castor oil is valued for its emollient properties. It is a common ingredient in lipsticks, lotions, and hair care products due to its moisturizing effects and ability to impart shine. The oil's natural origin and skin-friendly properties make it a popular choice among manufacturers aiming to create more natural and organic product lines.

Environmental Impact and Sustainability

One of the most significant advantages of castor oil is that it is derived from a renewable resource. The castor plant is cultivated in various regions around the world, with India being the largest producer. This plant is resilient and can grow in harsh conditions, reducing the need for extensive irrigation and chemical inputs.

Castor oil is biodegradable, meaning it breaks down naturally without leaving harmful residues in the environment. This characteristic makes it an environmentally friendly alternative to petroleum-based products. Its use in biodegradable lubricants and polymers helps reduce environmental pollution and dependence on non-renewable resources.

Despite its benefits, the sustainability of castor oil production faces challenges. The demand for castor oil has led to increased cultivation, which can sometimes result in land-use conflicts and mono-cropping practices. Sustainable agricultural practices, such as crop rotation and organic farming, are essential to mitigate these issues and ensure the long-term viability of castor oil production.

Integration into Conventional Medicine

Current Medical Applications

In conventional Western medicine, castor oil is primarily used as a potent laxative to treat occasional constipation. Castor oil's efficacy as a laxative is well-documented, and it is commonly recommended for short-term use.

It is also utilized in some dermatological treatments due to its antimicrobial and anti-inflammatory properties, which can help in treating conditions like acne and minor skin irritations. Additionally, castor oil is sometimes used in eye drops for its lubricating properties, aiding in the relief of dry eyes.

Challenges in Natural Ingredient Research

The lack of official research on castor oil is surprising given its long history of use and documented health benefits. This oversight highlights a significant gap in modern medical research, leaving castor oil's potential largely unexplored and undervalued in contemporary medicine.

The relationship between clinical studies and the convenience or interest in conducting them is complex, influenced by economic incentives, potential health benefits, scientific curiosity, and regulatory frameworks. Financial investment in clinical studies is substantial, covering laboratory facilities, clinical trials, personnel, and regulatory compliance. Pharmaceutical companies and stakeholders often seek a return on this investment, prioritizing projects that promise significant financial returns, such as new drugs or treatments that can be patented. Patents provide exclusive marketing rights, allowing companies to recoup their investment and make a profit, thus incentivizing research into novel pharmaceuticals and cutting-edge technologies.

Natural ingredients pose a unique challenge in this context. Many natural substances, including castor oil, have been used in traditional medicine for centuries and may offer therapeutic benefits. However, since natural ingredients cannot be patented, there is less financial incentive for pharmaceutical companies to invest in validating their efficacy. This lack of economic interest leads to underfunding and under-researching potentially beneficial natural treatments.

This economic focus creates a bias in the types of studies conducted. Preventative measures such as dietary changes, exercise, and public health campaigns do not offer the same profitability as pharmaceuticals, despite their potential to significantly improve public health outcomes.

However, not all medical research is driven by economic incentives. Academic institutions, government agencies, and non-profit organizations often fund studies based on scientific merit and public health needs rather than profitability. Increased funding for non-patentable research and a balanced approach to preventive and curative studies can ensure more holistic advancement of medical knowledge and public health.

Non-approved Uses of Medications

With all this in mind, it's important to recognize that traditional medicine often explores uses beyond official guidelines. In fact, modern medical practice involves "off-label" drug use, or non-approved uses of medications, demonstrating that treatments can be effective even without formal approval.

The use of drugs off-label refers to the prescription of medications for purposes other than those approved by regulatory agencies such as the U.S. Food and Drug Administration. This practice is legal and common in medical practice, particularly when there is evidence to support the safety and effectiveness of the medication for the off-label use.

For example, antidepressants are frequently prescribed off-label for anxiety disorders; antidepressants are also frequently prescribed off-label for insomnia[1]. Dermatologists often prescribe some oral antibiotics to treat acne due to their antimicrobial and anti-inflammatory properties, particularly when topical treatments are ineffective[2]. However, this off-label practice can negatively impact the microbiome, and excessive use of these antibiotics may contribute to antimicrobial resistance. The same conclusions apply to the frequent, unnecessary prescription of antibiotics for viral infections, such as the common cold or flu, even though antibiotics are intended solely for bacterial infections.

Here's what the FDA says about the off-label practice: "… healthcare providers generally may prescribe the drug for an unapproved use **when they judge that it is medically appropriate for their patient.**" [*Understanding Unapproved Use of Approved Drugs "Off Label"* (2018, February 5). U.S. Food and Drug Administration]

The Medicines and Healthcare products Regulatory Agency (MHRA), the equivalent of FDA for the United Kingdom, addresses to prescribers saying that "…before prescribing an unlicensed medicine or using a medicine off-label you should be satisfied that there is a **sufficient evidence base and/or experience of using the medicine to show its safety and efficacy**…" [*Off-label or unlicensed use of medicines: prescribers' responsibilities* (2014, December 11). GOV.UK.]

---

1   Everitt, H., Baldwin, D. S., Stuart, B., Lipinska, G., Mayers, A., Malizia, A. L., Manson, C. C., & Wilson, S. (2018). Antidepressants for insomnia in adults. *Cochrane Library*, 2018
2   Oral Antibiotic Treatment Options for Acne Vulgaris. (2020, October 12). JCAD | *The Journal of Clinical and Aesthetic Dermatology*

Well, castor oil, popular and well-documented over the years, demonstrates a broad experience of use, evidencing both safety and efficacy.

Despite the absence of formal regulatory endorsement, the beneficial effects of castor oil are widely recognized, they have been documented and trusted for centuries and should not deter us from utilizing it. Its extensive use in traditional medicine underscores its value in contemporary health practices. Embracing castor oil as a complementary treatment can offer holistic benefits, particularly when modern pharmaceuticals fall short.

While regulatory approval is important, the rich history and widespread anecdotal evidence supporting castor oil suggest that it remains a valuable resource in our health and wellness toolkit.

Castor Oil and Holistic Health in Modern Life

In today's fast-paced world, adopting a modern holistic approach to health is crucial. Our stressful lifestyles and poor dietary choices contribute to various health issues. Relying mainly on synthetic drugs offers temporary fixes rather than long-term solutions, often causing side effects and dependency.

A holistic approach considers the interconnectedness of mind, body, and spirit, promoting balance and overall wellness, acknowledging the impact of lifestyle, diet, mental state, and natural remedies. This approach builds a resilient foundation for health, enhancing the quality of life amidst modern demands.

The *fight-or-flight response*, triggered by stress, prepares our body for immediate action, causing alertness and tension, while the *rest-and-digest response*, activated during relaxation, promotes healing and recovery. Balancing these responses is essential, as chronic stress leads to health issues, while relaxation supports the body's restorative processes.

Natural remedies play a vital role by supporting the body's innate ability to heal and maintain balance, as they work synergistically with the body's systems. Castor oil is linked to holistic health through its multifaceted benefits that address both physical and mental well-being.

Physiological Healing Response

The rest-and-digest response is also known as the parasympathetic nervous system response.

When the parasympathetic nervous system is activated, it slows the heart rate, increases digestive activity, slows breathing, allowing for deeper breaths and improved oxygen exchange, and enhances immune response due to decreased stress hormone levels.

This state encourages the body to focus on processes that restore and maintain energy:

- **Healing**: in a relaxed state, the body's repair mechanisms function optimally. Cell regeneration and repair processes are enhanced, leading to faster healing of wounds and recovery from illnesses. The reduction of stress hormones like cortisol also decreases inflammation, further aiding in the healing process.
- **Digestion**: increased blood flow to the digestive organs facilitates nutrient absorption and effective digestion. Enzymes and digestive juices are secreted at optimal levels, ensuring food is broken down efficiently. This state prevents common digestive issues such as bloating, indigestion, and constipation.
- **Recovery**: during relaxation, the body diverts energy from external activities to internal maintenance. Muscle tension decreases, allowing muscles to recover from exertion and repair micro-tears. The nervous system's restoration also contributes to better mental clarity and emotional stability.

As we will explore further in the upcoming chapters, the effectiveness of the castor oil pack lies also in its ability to facilitate the transition from a state of stress to a state of relaxation.

CHAPTER 2
THE SCIENCE BEHIND CASTOR OIL

Botanical Origin: Castor Bean Plant

Plant Overview

The castor bean plant, known scientifically as Ricinus Communis, is a perennial flowering plant of the spurge family, Euphorbiaceae. Native to the southeastern Mediterranean Basin, India, and Eastern Africa, it has been cultivated in tropical and subtropical regions of the world due to its robust adaptability and the high demand for castor oil.

The plant features large, palmate leaves that can span up to 27 inches across. These leaves are typically deep green, but can sometimes exhibit hues of purple or red, depending on the variety. They resemble the shape of a hand, leading to the name "Palma Christi," or "Palm of Christ." This resemblance is linked to the plant's long-standing reputation for healing properties, reminiscent of the healing hands of Christ.

The stem of the plant ranges in color from reddish to purple, adding to its ornamental appeal.

The plant produces clusters of flowers, with female flowers situated at the top of the inflorescence, giving way to spiny, green seed pods. These seed pods contain the seeds, commonly referred to as beans, from which castor oil is extracted.

Growth and Cultivation Areas

Castor bean plants thrive in warm climates with full sun exposure. They prefer well-drained soils but are quite drought-tolerant, making them suitable for a variety of growing conditions. The primary cultivation regions include India, China, and Brazil, which are among the largest producers of castor oil globally.

The castor bean plant is not just valued for its oil but also plays a role in agriculture and ecology. It is often used in intercropping systems to improve soil health and reduce erosion. Its deep root system helps in soil aeration, and its foliage provides ground cover that minimizes weed growth.

Moreover, Ricinus communis has some allelopathic properties, meaning it can inhibit the growth of certain weeds and pests. This characteristic makes it a valuable plant in sustainable agriculture practices, where reducing chemical inputs is crucial.

While the castor bean plant is highly beneficial, it is important to note its toxic properties. The seeds contain ricin, a potent toxin that can be fatal if ingested. Therefore, handling and processing the seeds require careful management to ensure safety.

Despite its toxicity, castor oil extracted from the seeds is safe and has been used for centuries in medicine and cosmetics. The toxic protein ricin is not soluble in oil, and thus, castor oil itself is not toxic.

Extraction Methods

The extraction of castor oil from the seeds of the castor bean plant is a crucial process that determines the quality and properties of the final product.

Different processing methods also generate two different versions of castor oil in the market: Golden castor oil and Jamaican black castor oil. Golden castor oil is produced by cold-pressing fresh castor beans, resulting in a pale yellow oil that retains most of the natural nutrients without any added ingredients. Jamaican black castor oil, on the other hand, involves roasting the beans before extraction – they are boiled to extract the oil and so subjected to an intense amount of heat - which produces a much thicker, darker oil with ash content.

Cold Pressing

Cold pressing is a mechanical extraction method that involves pressing the castor beans without applying heat. This process is valued for its ability to preserve the natural qualities and beneficial compounds found in the oil.

The process consists of 4 phases:

- **Cleaning and Drying**: The castor beans are first cleaned to remove dirt and impurities. Then they are dried in order to reduce moisture content.
- **Crushing**: The dried beans are crushed to break open the seed coats and release the oil.
- **Pressing**: The crushed beans are then pressed using hydraulic or screw presses. During

this stage, the oil is extracted through mechanical pressure without the application of external heat.

- **Filtration**: The extracted oil is filtered to remove any remaining solid particles, resulting in a pure, high-quality oil.

Cold pressing preserves the natural compounds of castor oil. This method does not involve any chemicals, making the oil safer for medicinal and cosmetic uses. Cold-pressed oil retains more nutrients, antioxidants, and fatty acids, which are beneficial for skin, hair, and overall health. As a result, cold-pressed castor oil is often considered superior due to its purity and high nutrient content, making it ideal for applications in pharmaceuticals, cosmetics, and therapeutic treatments.

Another extraction method, often considered similar to cold pressing, is **expeller pressing**. The main difference between the two methods is temperature. Regular expeller pressing generates more heat from friction, potentially exposing the oil to temperatures up to 210°F, while cold pressing typically exposes the oil to temperatures up to 122°F. However, since castor oil must reach 230°F before it starts oxidizing and its nutrients break down, neither method damages the oil. Companies often choose expeller pressing over cold pressing because it extracts a higher percentage of oil from the seed, making the process more efficient and cost-effective.

Solvent Extraction Techniques

Solvent extraction involves using chemical solvents to dissolve and extract the oil from the castor beans. This method is commonly used for industrial purposes where large-scale oil production is required.

This kind of extraction can produce a higher yield of oil compared to cold pressing and is more economical for large-scale production, making it suitable for industrial applications. However, solvent-extracted castor oil may contain trace amounts of solvent, affecting its purity and suitability for certain applications. While effective for industrial uses, such as in the production of lubricants, plastics, and coatings, it may not be ideal for medicinal or cosmetic purposes where purity is paramount.

Chemical Composition

Castor oil is renowned for its unique chemical composition, which contributes to its wide range of health and therapeutic benefits. The primary component of castor oil is ricinoleic acid, a monounsaturated fatty acid that constitutes about 90% of the oil. This high concentration of ricinoleic acid is responsible for many of the oil's distinctive properties, because its molecular chain is highly versatile and easily modifiable.

Ricinoleic Acid

The low molecular weight and the presence of hydroxyl groups in ricinoleic acid enhance its skin permeability. The hydroxyl groups form hydrogen bonds with water molecules, increasing hydrophilicity and disrupting the lipid bilayers of the stratum corneum. This allows ricinoleic acid to penetrate more deeply into the skin, facilitating systemic absorption and effectiveness of castor oil throughout the body.

This deep absorption is due to the unique chemical composition of ricinoleic acid that has a molecular weight of approximately 298.46 Daltons[3], so that it is able to filter through the lower layer of the epidermis and reach the areas where blood and lymphatic vessels reside.

Lymphatic vessels are generally located just below the skin's surface, typically within a range of about 0.3 to 1.5 inches (approximately 0.8 to 3.8 centimeters) deep. Blood vessels under the skin, particularly veins and capillaries, are generally located quite close to the surface. Typically, they can be found within a few millimeters to about 0.4 inches (approximately 1 centimeter) deep.

The unique features of ricinoleic acid impart several beneficial properties. Some of the most popular are:

Anti-inflammatory properties: ricinoleic acid is known for its potent anti-inflammatory effects. It works by inhibiting the release of certain inflammatory mediators, making it effective in reducing swelling, pain, and redness in various conditions such as arthritis and muscle aches.

Antimicrobial activity: ricinoleic acid exhibits antimicrobial properties against a variety of bacteria, viruses, and fungi. This makes castor oil useful for treating skin infections, acne, and even minor wounds.

Moisturizing and emollient: the structure of ricinoleic acid allows it to penetrate deeply into the skin, providing intense hydration and acting as an emollient. It helps to lock in moisture, making it highly effective in treating dry and sensitive skin.

---

3   Bos, J. D., & Meinardi, M. M. H. M. (2000). The 500 Dalton rule for the skin penetration of chemical compounds and drugs. *Experimental Dermatology, 9*(3), 165–169

Nature's Transporter

Castor oil is considered an excellent carrier oil due to its specific chemical structure and molecular weight, making it highly effective for this purpose. Its unique properties enable it to deliver medications into the body more quickly and efficiently[4], and this advantage extends to essential oils as well.

Here are some applications in which castor oil is frequently used as a carrier agent:

- **Aromatherapy and essential oils**: castor oil is an excellent carrier oil for diluting essential oils before topical application and transporting them through the skin to enhance their absorption.
- **Medicinal and therapeutic treatments**: in traditional and alternative medicine, castor oil is used as a carrier for other medicinal agents due to its ability to penetrate deeply into the skin and deliver active ingredients efficiently to the targeted area.
- **Skincare products**: castor oil is often included in lotions, creams, and ointments as a carrier oil to deliver active ingredients such as vitamins, antioxidants, and other beneficial compounds into the skin. Its moisturizing and emollient properties also enhance the effectiveness of skincare products.
- **Hair care treatments**: in hair care, castor oil serves as a carrier oil for essential oils and other hair growth-promoting ingredients. It helps in moisturizing the scalp, reinforcing hair follicles, and stimulating healthy hair growth.
- **Massage therapy**: castor oil is used as a base oil in massage therapy, carrying essential oils and other therapeutic agents that can help relieve muscle tension, reduce inflammation, and promote relaxation.
- **Topical pain relief**: castor oil is used as a carrier in pain relief balms and liniments, helping to deliver anti-inflammatory and analgesic compounds through the skin to alleviate joint and muscle pain.

By serving as a carrier agent in these various applications, castor oil enhances the delivery and effectiveness of active ingredients, making it a versatile and valuable component in both traditional and modern therapeutic practices.

Other Components

Besides ricinoleic acid, castor oil contains several other components that enhance its properties:

---

4   Shikanov, A., Vaisman, B., Krasko, M. Y., Nyska, A., & Domb, A. J. (2004). Poly(sebacic acid-co-ricinoleic acid) biodegradable carrier for paclitaxel: In vitro release and in vivo toxicity. *Journal of Biomedical Materials Research. Part A*, 69A(1), 47–54.

Oleic Acid: this monounsaturated fatty acid makes up about 2-6% of castor oil. It contributes to the oil's emollient properties and aids in skin hydration (it is found in olive oil, for example).

Linoleic Acid: also present in small amounts, about 1-5% linoleic acid is a polyunsaturated omega-6 fatty acid (also found in sesame oil). It is essential for maintaining the skin's barrier function and reducing inflammation.

Stearic Acid: this saturated fatty acid is found in minor quantities in castor oil. It provides moisturizing benefits and helps to improve the texture and stability of cosmetic formulations.

Palmitic Acid: another saturated fatty acid, palmitic acid has emollient properties that help to soften and smooth the skin.

Vitamin E: castor oil contains vitamin E, a powerful antioxidant that protects the skin from oxidative stress and helps to maintain skin health by reducing the signs of aging.

Minerals and Other Phytochemicals: trace amounts of minerals and various phytochemicals in castor oil contribute to its overall therapeutic profile. These compounds can enhance skin health and support the body's natural healing processes.

The combination of these components in castor oil results in a synergistic effect, amplifying its efficacy in various applications. The high concentration of ricinoleic acid, coupled with other fatty acids and bioactive compounds, makes castor oil a versatile and powerful natural remedy.

Unsuspected Activity of Castor Oil

Ricinoleic acid is renowned for its unique ability to mimic prostaglandins, a group of physiologically active lipid compounds. This ability underpins many of the therapeutic effects attributed to castor oil. To understand how ricinoleic acid achieves this, it's essential to delve into the structure and function of prostaglandins.

Strategic Lipid Compounds

Prostaglandins are lipid molecules produced enzymatically from fatty acids. They are found in virtually all tissues and organs and are produced by almost all nucleated cells.

Prostaglandins resemble hormones as they regulate various functions in your body, instruct-

ing it on what actions to take and when. They are produced by human tissues at the site of injury, damage, or infection[5].

To carry out their roles effectively, prostaglandins interact intricately with both lipid membranes and specific receptors within the body.

Lipid membranes form the boundary between the inside of a cell and its external environment, playing a critical role in maintaining their integrity and functionality. The unique composition and properties of lipid membranes allow them to serve as barriers, facilitate communication and transport, and maintain the overall integrity and state of balance of cells.

Receptors are specialized protein molecules located on the surface of or inside cells. They act as binding sites for signaling molecules, such as hormones, neurotransmitters, or drugs, allowing these molecules to exert their effects on the cell. When a signaling molecule binds to its receptor, it triggers a specific response within the cell, which can involve changes in cellular activity, function, or behavior.

The interaction of prostaglandin with lipid membranes and receptors is crucial for the signaling processes that enable it to regulate various physiological functions.

The capacity of the same prostaglandin to either stimulate or inhibit a reaction depends on the type of receptor it binds to in different tissues[6].

Prostaglandins have diverse and significant roles in the body, here are their primary functions:

- **Inflammation and Pain:** prostaglandins are involved as mediators in the inflammatory response, contributing to the swelling, redness, and pain associated with inflammation. They increase the sensitivity of nerve endings, making the sensation of pain more pronounced.
- **Regulation of Blood Flow**: prostaglandins can cause blood vessels to dilate (vasodilation), increasing blood flow to specific areas. This is crucial in controlling blood pressure and responding to injury or infection.
- **Formation of Blood Clots:** some prostaglandins promote the clumping together of platelets, aiding in the formation of blood clots and preventing excessive bleeding.
- **Gastrointestinal Protection:** prostaglandins stimulate the secretion of mucus and bicarbonate in the stomach lining, which protects the stomach from acidic damage.
- **Reproductive Functions:** prostaglandins play a role in inducing labor by stimulating uterine contractions. They are also involved in the regulation of the ovulation, the menstrual cycle and the shedding of the uterine lining.

5   Professional, C. C. M. (n.d.). Prostaglandins. *Cleveland Clinic*
6   Prostaglandin. (2024, May 16). *Wikipedia*

- **Kidney Function:** prostaglandins help regulate blood flow within the kidneys, influencing the filtration rate and the balance of water and electrolytes.
- **Immune System Modulation:** they can modulate the immune response by affecting the activity of various immune cells, thereby influencing how the body responds to infections and other immune challenges.
- **Bronchial Functions:** prostaglandins can cause the contraction or relaxation of smooth muscle in the airways, impacting respiratory functions and conditions like asthma.

Structural Facts

The key to understanding how ricinoleic acid acts is to recognize its similarity to prostaglandins.

Ricinoleic acid is an unsaturated omega-9 fatty acid and it is structurally similar to prostaglandins, both featuring a hydroxyl group on the 12th carbon atom.

Ricinoleic Acid structure   Prostaglandin structure

At the core of every prostaglandin molecule is a five-membered ring with oxygen atoms at specific positions, giving prostaglandins their reactivity and unique chemical properties. This ring forms the basis for classifying prostaglandins into different types and functions, as mentioned in the previous paragraph.

The structural similarity allows ricinoleic acid to mimic the action of prostaglandins and influence similar biological processes, particularly in reducing inflammation and pain. By acknowledging these molecular similarities, we can better understand the mechanisms through which castor oil and its active components exert their therapeutic effects.

Mechanisms of Action

Receptor Binding: Ricinoleic acid can interact with the same receptors of prostaglandins, either by directly binding to them or by influencing the lipid environment of the cell membrane, thereby modulating the receptors' activity.

Inflammation Modulation: one of the primary roles of prostaglandins is the modulation of inflammation. Ricinoleic acid has been shown to have a significant anti-inflammatory effect[78], which is partly due to its ability to mimic the action of anti-inflammatory prostaglandins. It reduces the synthesis of pro-inflammatory cytokines and mediators, thereby helping to control inflammation and associated pain.

Smooth Muscle Regulation: smooth muscle is found in various organs and structures within the body. Smooth muscle is found in the walls of hollow organs such as the intestines, stomach, bladder, and uterus. In blood and lymph vessels (excluding capillaries), it is referred to as vascular smooth muscle. Additionally, smooth muscle is present in the tracts of the urinary, respiratory, and reproductive systems[9]. Prostaglandins play a crucial role in regulating the contraction and relaxation of smooth muscle tissue, such as that found in the intestines and uterus. Ricinoleic acid can mimic these effects, which explains its use as a natural laxative and in facilitating labor.

Systemic Effects and Benefits

Here are the widespread effects on the human body and the pain-relieving properties it can have.

1. **Anti-Inflammatory and Analgesic Properties**: we will dive into these properties in Chapter 3.
2. **Immune System Modulation:** we will dive into these properties in Chapter 3.
3. **Gastrointestinal Benefits:** we will dive into these properties in Chapter 3.
4. **Skin and Hair Health:** we will dive into these properties in Chapter 4 and Chapter 5.
5. **Hormonal Balance and Reproductive Health:** we will dive into these properties in Chapter 6.

---

7   Vieira, C., Evangelista, S., Cirillo, R., Lippi, A., Maggi, C. A., & Manzini, S. (2000b). Effect of ricinoleic acid in acute and subchronic experimental models of inflammation. *Mediators of Inflammation*, 9(5), 223–228

8   Boddu, S. H., Alsaab, H., Umar, S., Bonam, S. P., Gupta, H., & Ahmed, S. (2015). Anti-inflammatory effects of a novel ricinoleic acid poloxamer gel system for transdermal delivery. *International Journal of Pharmaceutics*, 479(1), 207–211

9   Smooth muscle. (2024, May 26). Wikipedia.

CHAPTER 3
HEALTH BENEFITS OF CASTOR OIL

Digestive Health

Digestive health refers to the proper functioning of the digestive system, which includes the stomach, intestines, and related organs that help in the breakdown, absorption, and assimilation of nutrients from food.

Problems in digestive health can lead to a variety of other health issues throughout the body due to the interconnected nature of bodily systems, such as **poor nutrient absorption**, **weakening of the immune system** (a large part of the immune system is situated in the gut itself), **inflammation** both in the digestive tract and systemically, **mental health conditioning** (the gut-brain axis is a critical communication pathway), **hormonal imbalance** (the gut is involved in the metabolism and excretion of hormones), **accumulation of toxins**.

Relieving Constipation

Castor oil has been used for centuries as a natural remedy for constipation due to its potent laxative properties. Ricinoleic acid promotes the stimulation of intestinal peristalsis and water retention in the intestine.

Stimulation of intestinal peristalsis is the mechanism that starts when ricinoleic acid binds to EP3 prostanoid receptors, which are part of the prostaglandin receptor family[10]. This activation results in the contraction of smooth muscle cells in the intestinal wall, and this enhances the wave-like contractions that propel contents through the intestines promoting bowel movements and relieving constipation.

Water retention in the intestine happens because, similar to prostaglandins, ricinoleic acid increases the secretion of water and electrolytes (such as chloride ions, sodium - Na^+ - and

---

10   Tunaru, S., Althoff, T. F., Nüsing, R. M., Diener, M., & Offermanns, S. (2012). *Castor oil induces laxation and uterus contraction via ricinoleic acid activating prostaglandin EP 3 receptors.* Proceedings of the National Academy of Sciences of the United States of America, 109(23), 9179–9184.

potassium - K$^+$). These minerals carry an electric charge and help regulate the distribution of water in and out of cells and tissues. This increase in the overall ionic concentration in the intestine, in turn draws more water into the lumen via osmosis.

The combined effect of increased water and electrolyte secretion from castor oil softens the stool, making it bulkier and easier to pass.

USAGE GUIDELINES

To use castor oil as a laxative, it is typically ingested orally. The oil is available in both liquid form and as capsules. Here are guidelines for its use[11]:

Adults: usually 15 ml (1 tablespoon) to 60 ml (4 tablespoons). This can vary based on individual needs and the severity of constipation.

Children aged 2-12 years: a lower dose of 5 to 15 ml is suggested (1 to 3 teaspoons). It is crucial to consult a healthcare provider before giving castor oil to children.

For quicker results, it is advisable to take castor oil on an empty stomach. Effects typically occur within 2 to 6 hours after ingestion.

Castor oil can have a strong, unpleasant taste, so mixing it with a small amount of juice or a flavored beverage can help mask it. Some people prefer to take it as a chilled shot or use capsules to avoid the taste altogether.

Gut Health made Gentler

For addressing constipation, while oral consumption may provide immediate relief, it often leads to an urgent and uncomfortable need to use the bathroom. A more holistic approach focuses on regulating gut function and environment for long-term health. Castor oil packs are an effective method, gently stimulating the gut without causing harsh urgency, fostering natural and sustainable digestive health improvements.

In pursuing overall health, the goal should be to naturally enhance the body's function without overstimulation. Castor oil packs offer more benefits than just laxation. Oral consumption primarily provides a laxative effect, but does not significantly impact inflammation or microbiome balance. Additionally, relaxation is crucial for effective colon cleansing, liver detox, and lymphatic drainage. Castor oil packs are preferred because they support colon cleansing and improve bowel movements as effectively as oral laxatives but without causing cramping. And last but not least, they help shift the body into a relaxed state, promoting natural detoxification, cleansing, and microbiome balance.

---

11   *Castor Oil Dosage Guide + Max Dose*, Adjustments. (n.d.). Drugs.com

Gut microbiome imbalance can result from yeast overgrowth like Candida albicans, which ferments sugars into alcohol and acetaldehyde, causing hangover-like symptoms. Factors like antibiotic use, birth control pills, and estrogen dominance contribute to this condition.

Managing it involves balancing the gut microbiome through probiotics, a low-sugar diet, and the use of castor oil packs, which can significantly help.

Castor oil packs reduce inflammation and make the environment less hospitable for the growth of yeast such as Candida albicans[12]. Studies in mice show that castor oil stimulates contractility and peristalsis via PGE3 receptors on smooth muscle[13], and also supports nitric oxide production in the intestine[14], enhancing circulatory flow and providing protective mechanisms like antimicrobial actions[15] and biofilm breakdown. Biofilm is a protective layer that bad bacteria produce to shield themselves from being eliminated, making it difficult to maintain a balanced microbiome. Castor oil can break down that barrier, allowing harmful bacteria to be eradicated from the gut and beneficial bacteria to survive.

The packs also promote nutrient absorption and reduce inflammation, being rich in Omega 6 and 9, vitamin E, and polyphenols, which support overall gut health.

For more in-depth information on how to use castor oil packs you can refer to Chapter 7.

Pain Relief and Anti-Inflammatory Properties

Joint Pain and Arthritis

Joint pain can result from a variety of causes, including injury, inflammation, and chronic wear and tear. Arthritis, on the other hand, is a more specific condition characterized by inflammation of the joints. There are more than a hundred types of arthritis, with rheumatoid arthritis and osteoarthritis being the most common.

---

12 Valera, M. C., Maekawa, L. E., De Oliveira, L. D., Jorge, A. O. C., Shygei, R., & Carvalho, C. a. T. (2013). In vitro antimicrobial activity of auxiliary chemical substances and natural extracts on Candida albicans and Enterococcus faecalis in root canals. *Journal of Applied Oral Science, 21*(2), 118–123.

13 Tunaru, S., Althoff, T. F., Nüsing, R. M., Diener, M., & Offermanns, S. (2012b). Castor oil induces laxation and uterus contraction via ricinoleic acid activating prostaglandin EP 3 receptors. *Proceedings of the National Academy of Sciences of the United States of America, 109*(23), 9179–9184

14 Mascolo, N., Izzo, A. A., Autore, G., Barbato, F., & Capasso, F. (1994, January 1). Nitric oxide and castor oil-induced diarrhea. *Journal of Pharmacology and Experimental Therapeutics.*

15 Stasko, N., McHale, K., Hollenbach, S. J., Martin, M., & Doxey, R. (2018). Nitric Oxide-Releasing Macromolecule Exhibits Broad-Spectrum Antifungal Activity and Utility as a Topical Treatment for Superficial Fungal Infections. *Antimicrobial Agents and Chemotherapy, 62*(7)

Symptoms often include swelling, stiffness, decreased range of motion, and varying degrees of pain, which can significantly affect one's quality of life.

APPLICATION METHODS AND EFFECTIVENESS

Castor oil has been traditionally used to alleviate joint pain and arthritis.

The anti-inflammatory properties of ricinoleic acid help reduce swelling and pain, while the oil's high viscosity allows it to stay on the skin longer, providing prolonged relief. It works by activating EP3 prostanoid receptors, which are involved in inflammatory pathways, and regulating the immune response by decreasing the production of pro-inflammatory cytokines and mediators[16].

Here's a detailed look at how castor oil can be applied and its effectiveness in treating them.

Direct massage: you can start by warming a small amount of castor oil in your hands, and then gently massage the oil into the affected joints for about 5-10 minutes. This helps improve circulation and allows the oil to penetrate deeply into the tissues.

Castor oil packs: cover the painful joint with a castor oil pack, and place a heating pad or hot water bottle on top[17]. Leave it on for 30-60 minutes. This method enhances the absorption of ricinoleic acid and provides sustained relief.

For more in-depth information on how to use castor oil packs you can refer to Chapter 7.

Combination with essential oils: mix castor oil with essential oils like lavender or peppermint, which have additional anti-inflammatory and analgesic properties, and apply the mixture to the affected areas for enhanced pain relief.

In these cases, consistency is key: applying castor oil packs on joint pain at least three times a week for four weeks can address both the short-term and long-term benefits of this treatment. Incorporating castor oil massage into the daily routine is even better for arthritis, over a period of a few months, to achieve a marked decrease in inflammation and pain.

---

16   Vieira, C., Evangelista, S., Cirillo, R., Lippi, A., Maggi, C. A., & Manzini, S. (2000b). Effect of ricinoleic acid in acute and subchronic experimental models of inflammation. Mediators of Inflammation, 9(5), 223–228 | Boddu, S. H., Alsaab, H., Umar, S., Bonam, S. P., Gupta, H., & Ahmed, S. (2015). Anti-inflammatory effects of a novel ricinoleic acid poloxamer gel system for transdermal delivery. International Journal of Pharmaceutics, 479(1), 207–211

17   Dr.Sahbanathul Missiriya, S.Sylvia Deva Roopa (2015, September). Effectiveness of castor oil massage with hot application on knee joint pain among women. *International Journal of Innovative Research in Technology*

Muscle Aches and Pains

Muscle aches and pains, also known as myalgia, can arise from various factors, including overuse, tension, or minor injuries. Castor oil offers a natural remedy to alleviate these discomforts.

TECHNIQUES FOR RELIEF AND EFFECTIVENESS

One of the simplest methods to relieve muscle pain with castor oil is through direct **topical application**. Slightly heat the castor oil to enhance its absorption into the skin by placing the bottle in warm water for a few minutes. (Never put castor oil in the microwave.) Apply generously by massaging the warm oil onto the affected area in circular motions to ensure deep penetration, then cover the area with a soft cloth to keep the oil in place and retain warmth. Let the oil sit for at least an hour, or overnight for optimal results. This technique helps in reducing inflammation and provides a soothing effect on sore muscles.

Castor oil packs are another highly effective method for relieving muscle pain. This technique is particularly beneficial for larger areas of muscle discomfort. Place a heating pad or hot water bottle over the pack because the heat helps in deeper penetration of the oil. Leave the pack on for 45 minutes to an hour, use this time to relax and allow the oil to work its magic.

Castor oil packs are known to enhance circulation, reduce inflammation, and promote healing.

For widespread muscle aches, a **castor oil bath** can be a soothing remedy: add a few tablespoons of castor oil to a warm bath and then immerse yourself in the bath for 20-30 minutes. While soaking, gently massage any particularly sore areas. This method allows for full-body relaxation and relief, perfect for conditions like fibromyalgia or general muscle soreness after intense physical activity.

The efficacy of castor oil in treating muscle aches and pains is supported by various studies highlighting its anti-inflammatory and analgesic properties. As already has been said, ricinoleic acid inhibits the production of inflammatory markers such as prostaglandins and cytokines, which are often elevated in muscle pain and soreness.

In various animal studies, castor oil was compared to capsaicin. Capsaicin is a key ingredient in creams and patches that provide pain relief. When applied to your skin, it helps block pain messages from reaching your nerves[18]. Castor oil was found to be equally effective in reducing inflammation and swelling but, unlike capsaicin, it did not cause irritating redness.

It works by stimulating the lymphatic system and reducing pain perception by decreasing

---

18   Altınterim, B. (2013). Cayenne, Capsaicin and Substance-P. *ResearchGate*.

substance P, which is a neurotransmitter involved in pain signaling[19]. This mechanism is similar to acupuncture and explains why castor oil packs are commonly used for treating arthritic joints, sprains, and strains.

Besides, castor oil's ability to enhance blood circulation to the area, via nitric oxide[20], also contributes to its effectiveness in treating muscle pain. Improved circulation helps in delivering oxygen and nutrients to the affected muscles, accelerating the healing process.

Immune System Support

The immune system protects the body from infections and diseases by identifying and neutralizing harmful pathogens. A proper detoxification of the body is fundamental for the immune system's function, through the removal of waste and toxins from bodily tissues. The body's detoxification system involves several organs that work together, such as the liver, the intestines, the colon, the lungs and the lymphatic system, which also plays a direct role in immune function.

Toxic compounds and incomplete body detoxification can exert pro-inflammatory effects and disrupt hormonal or metabolic balance, in addition to promoting oxidative stress. In short, they hinder the normal functioning of cells and physiological processes.

Castor oil packs are used to support immune system health through several mechanisms related to:

Inflammation reduction: by reducing inflammation in the body, castor oil packs can help lower the burden on the immune system, because chronic inflammation can impair the immune response, increasing the body's vulnerability to infections and diseases.

Improving circulation: castor oil packs increase blood flow to the applied area. Enhanced circulation can help deliver nutrients and oxygen more efficiently to tissues and organs, supporting overall immune function. Good circulation is vital for maintaining the health and function of the immune system.

Promoting relaxation and stress reduction: the application of castor oil packs induces a relaxation response by activating the parasympathetic nervous system. This helps to lower stress levels, which can otherwise suppress the immune response.

---

19   Vieira, C., Evangelista, S., Cirillo, R., Lippi, A., Maggi, C. A., & Manzini, S. (2000b). Effect of ricinoleic acid in acute and subchronic experimental models of inflammation. *Mediators of Inflammation*, 9(5), 223–228

20   Ricinoleic acid, the active ingredient of Castor oil, increases nitric oxide synthase activity in the rat ileum and colon | *Health & Environmental Research Online* | US EPA. (n.d.).

Detoxification and **lymphatic circulation enhancement**: let's delve deeper into these mechanisms in the following paragraphs.

Detoxification and the liver

The liver is a critical organ for detoxification, as it acts as the body's primary filter, processing blood from the digestive tract before it circulates to the rest of the body and detoxifies chemicals. This ensures that harmful substances are identified and neutralized before they can cause damage.

A common anecdotal experience is waking up between 1 and 3 AM, often accompanied by night sweats, hot flashes, the need to use the bathroom, or feeling thirsty. According to Traditional Chinese Medicine, this time corresponds to the liver's peak detoxification period. The liver is working hard to process and eliminate toxins from the body, which can disrupt sleep and cause these symptoms. Recognizing this pattern can help understand the importance of supporting liver health for detoxification and better sleep quality.

The liver produces bile, a digestive fluid that is stored in the gallbladder and released into the small intestine, where it aids in digestion and carries waste products for elimination. The liver also helps regulate blood composition and it stores essential nutrients and releases them into the blood as needed, ensuring that the body has a steady supply of energy and nutrients.

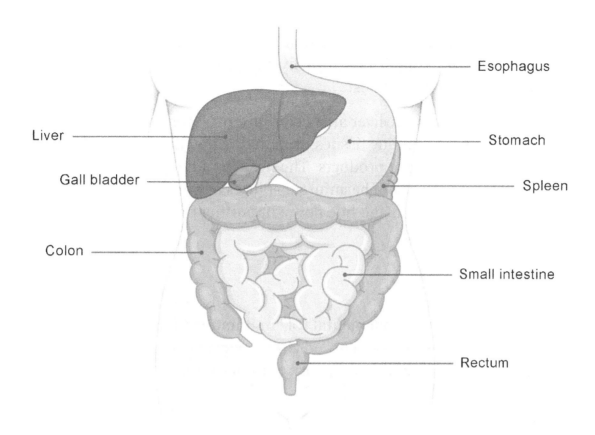

Liver detoxification is crucial for three fundamental reasons:

1. **Toxin Neutralization**: The liver neutralizes a wide range of toxins, including environmental pollutants, alcohol, medications, and metabolic byproducts. By converting these substances into less harmful compounds, the liver protects other organs and tissues from damage.
2. **Immune Support**: The liver contains a large number of immune cells which capture and digest bacteria, old blood cells, and other debris from the bloodstream. This helps to maintain a healthy immune system and prevents infections.
3. **Hormone Regulation**: The liver helps regulate hormone levels by breaking down and removing excess hormones from the bloodstream. This includes hormones such as insulin, estrogen, and cortisol, which are crucial for maintaining hormonal balance and overall health.

CASTOR OIL PACKS APPLICATION

As the liver plays a crucial role as the master detoxifying organ, castor oil packs for immune health are preferably applied to this organ to lower inflammation and to detox the body.

Castor oil packs help to detoxify the body thanks to its chemical characteristics. Not only does it promote glutathione[21], the body's primary detoxification agent, but it also provides fat-soluble nutrients such as vitamin E and omega 6 and 9 fatty acids. Additionally, it boosts nitric oxide[22], which plays a significant role in liver regeneration[23]. This combination delivers a robust and healthy antioxidant boost.

Applying castor oil packs over the liver area helps improve liver function by reducing inflammation in the liver and surrounding tissues, stimulating the lymphatic system, and aiding in the drainage of toxins and waste products. The heat from the pack encourages blood flow, helping to break down and flush out harmful substances more effectively. Additionally, castor oil packs help enhance digestion and bile flow, supporting the liver's role in processing and metabolizing nutrients and fats.

Lymphatic Circulation

The lymphatic system plays a fundamental role in immune function and consists of a large network that includes lymphatic vessels and lymph nodes. Lymph nodes filter the lymph to identify and fight infection, while the network of tubules transports white blood cells (lymphocytes) and collects waste from tissues.

Many of the lymphatic vessels sit just under the surface of our skin, typically within a range of about 0.3 to 1.5 inches (approximately 0.8 to 3.8 centimeters) deep. However, the exact depth can vary depending on the specific area of the body and individual anatomical differences. In some areas, particularly near joints and in the extremities, lymphatic vessels may be closer to the surface, while in others, they may be slightly deeper.

After being collected and filtered, waste is transported to the bloodstream for elimination, a process known as lymphatic drainage. When the lymphatic system malfunctions, waste and toxins can accumulate, leading to illness.

21   Holm, T., Brøgger-Jensen, M. R., Johnson, L., & Kessel, L. (2013). Glutathione Preservation during Storage of Rat Lenses in Optisol-GS and Castor Oil. *PloS One*, 8(11), e79620

22   Ricinoleic acid, the active ingredient of Castor oil, increases nitric oxide synthase activity in the rat ileum and colon | *Health & Environmental Research Online* | US EPA. (n.d.).

23   Iwakiri, Y., & Kim, M. Y. (2015). Nitric oxide in liver diseases. *Trends in Pharmacological Sciences*, 36(8), 524–536.

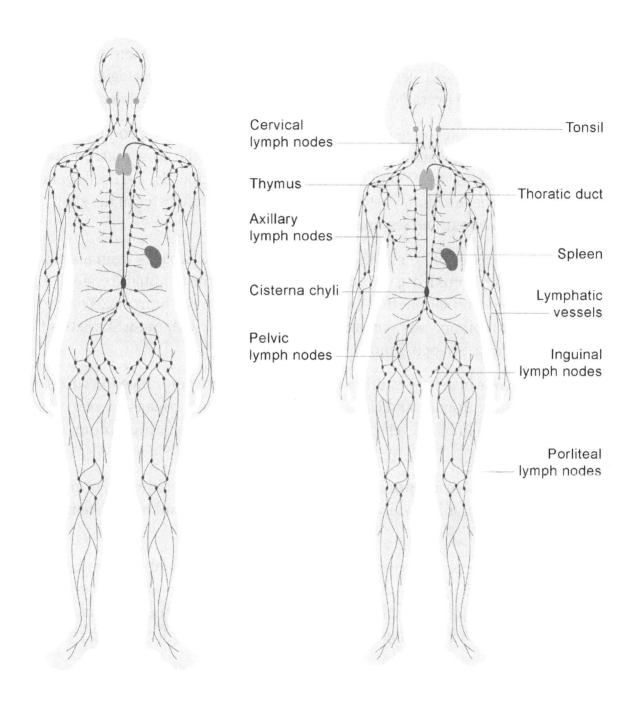

Cervical
lymph nodes

Thymus

Axillary
lymph nodes

Cisterna chyli

Pelvic
lymph nodes

Tonsil

Thoratic duct

Spleen

Lymphatic
vessels

Inguinal
lymph nodes

Porliteal
lymph nodes

The Lymphatic System - Lymphocytes, the immune system's disease-fighting cells, are primarily produced and stored in lymphatic tissues such as the thymus gland (in your upper chest behind your breastbone or sternum), spleen (a small organ inside your left rib cage, near the stomach), lymph nodes (small, bean-shaped organs that filter substances), and the lymphatic tissue lining the small intestine known as Peyer's patches or aggregated lymphatic follicles. The lymphatic system is a highly intricate network that collaborates closely with both the blood circulatory system (the liver is the organ responsible for filtering and detoxifying the blood) and the digestive system (the small intestine).

TECHNIQUES AND EFFECTIVENESS

The prevailing hypothesis on how castor oil enhances the immune system is suggested by a study that indicates it increases T-cell activity[24] in the skin and boosts prostaglandin levels. This rise in T-11 cells signifies an overall enhancement in the body's specific defense mechanisms.

In fact, lymphocytes are categorized into B-cells and T-cells. B-cells produce antibodies to combat bacteria and toxins, whereas T-cells, which develop in the bone marrow and thymus gland, target and destroy viruses, fungi, and cancer cells. Specifically, T-11 cells generate antibodies vital for immune function. Castor oil stimulates T-lymphocytes in the skin, initiating a localized and systemic immune response.

A specific way to use castor oil to enhance lymphatic function derives from an old practice called dry brushing. **Dry brushing** mechanically stimulates the lymphatic system, exfoliates the skin, and improves circulation, that's why it's best done in the morning. You can apply a small amount of castor oil on your skin and use a body brush with natural bristles to gently exfoliate the skin in long, sweeping motions toward the heart.

Using castor oil in your brushing routine not only helps with tolerance but also enhances the movement of your lymphatic and circulatory systems. This is because castor oil supports smooth muscle function in blood vessels and the lymphatic system, promoting better circulation and lymphatic flow.

For immune support, **castor oil packs** are beneficial as they stimulate the lymphatic system and reduce inflammation, all of which contribute to a stronger and more efficient immune response.

Castor oil packs are often placed **over the liver** (right side of the abdomen, under the ribcage), in **key lymphatic areas** such as the upper abdomen, **on the gut**, or even on the thymus gland, which is a part of the lymphatic system, located in the upper chest. They can be used several times a week (ranging from once to daily), typically for 30 to 60 minutes each session, at least.

For more in-depth information on how to use castor oil packs you can refer to Chapter 7.

Thyroid

The thyroid and immune system are closely interconnected, meaning that thyroid problems can influence the immune system, and vice versa.

---

24   Grady H. Immunomodulation through Castor Oil Packs. *Journal of Naturopathic Medicine.* 1998;7(1):84-89.

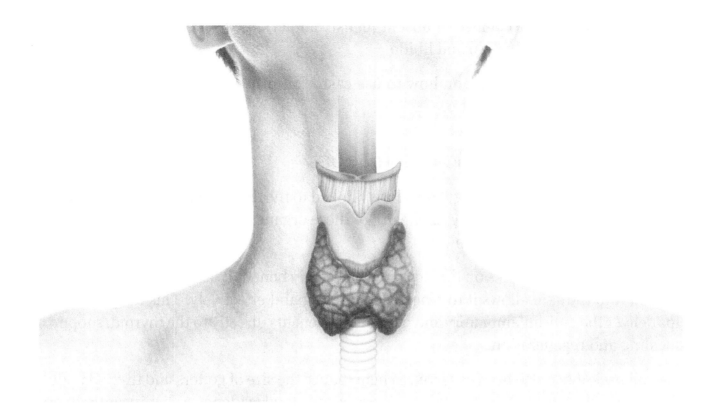

In thyroid autoimmune disease, the immune system mistakenly targets healthy tissues, leading to inflammation and eventually chronic damage. This can result in the thyroid gland producing insufficient thyroid hormone (hypothyroidism) or an excess of it (hyperthyroidism).

Also proper functioning of the lymphatic system is crucial for managing autoimmune responses and supporting overall thyroid health. If the lymphatic system is compromised or sluggish, it can contribute to a buildup of toxins that might exacerbate autoimmune responses, including those affecting the thyroid. Chronic inflammation, common in autoimmune diseases, can affect both the lymphatic system and the thyroid.

The thyroid gland plays a fundamental role in regulating various bodily functions and is interconnected with multiple organs like the heart, the brain, the muscles, the bones, the skin, and in particular with the following systems:

- **the liver** which metabolizes thyroid hormones, converting the inactive form (T4) to the active form (T3). Thyroid function directly affects liver metabolism, and liver diseases can impact thyroid hormone levels;
- **the digestive system**, as thyroid hormones influence metabolism and digestive function. Hypothyroidism can slow digestion, leading to constipation, while hyperthyroidism can speed up digestion, causing diarrhea;
- **the reproductive system** as thyroid hormones are crucial for reproductive health. In women, hypothyroidism can cause irregular menstrual cycles and infertility, while hyper-

thyroidism can lead to lighter or absent menstrual periods. In men, thyroid imbalances can affect sperm production and libido.

For more in-depth information on how to use castor oil packs on the thyroid for hormone balance you can refer to Chapter 6.

CASTOR OIL AND APPLICATION TECHNIQUES

As we have learned, the liver and gut are closely linked to the thyroid, along with the lymphatic system. Consequently, supporting the health of these organs through **castor oil packs** also promotes proper thyroid function.

Additionally, castor oil packs on the thyroid can directly benefit it, as the deep penetration of castor oil into the skin allows it to reach the thyroid gland effectively. This deep absorption helps deliver the anti-inflammatory and detoxifying benefits directly to the thyroid, supporting its healing and regeneration.

Castor oil packs have also been observed to help reduce the size of goiters and thyroid nodules. Although not claiming complete removal, there is anecdotal evidence of significant reduction in size when using the packs regularly.

Regular use of castor oil packs can help balance hormones and alleviate various symptoms associated with thyroid disorders, such as neck pain, swelling, and discomfort. The soothing effect of the warm castor oil pack provides relief from these physical symptoms, thereby improving overall comfort and well-being.

However, it is important to note that when using castor oil packs in the presence of thyroid issues, precautions are necessary due to the thyroid's susceptibility to changes in the body. Even a detoxification boost can lead to imbalances in the delicate body system. Therefore, any practice involving the thyroid should be gradual and implemented over a period of time, with careful precautions and thoughtful consideration.

Targeting the liver: when used on the liver, regular castor oil packs can help in balancing hormones by supporting liver function. The liver plays a crucial role in metabolizing hormones, including those produced by the thyroid. Thyroid function directly affects liver metabolism, and liver diseases can impact thyroid hormone levels. By enhancing liver detoxification, castor oil indirectly supports hormonal balance, which is vital for thyroid health.

Targeting the thyroid: castor oil packs can also be done directly on the thyroid. For thyroid health, a castor oil pack is applied directly over the thyroid gland. This involves soaking a piece of flannel in castor oil, placing it on the thyroid area, and covering it with a heat source to enhance absorption, typically for one hour. You can repeat two or three times a week, or even once a day. The deep penetration of castor oil helps deliver the anti-inflammatory and detoxifying benefits directly to it, supporting its healing and regeneration. This is applicable to both men and women.

Best practice: target both of them! When using castor oil packs for liver detoxification, a recommended and beneficial practice is to protect the thyroid at the same time. In fact detoxification mobilizes toxins, and the thyroid is highly susceptible to heavy metals and various toxins. Applying a castor oil pack to the thyroid while using one on the liver can help reduce inflammation and potential damage, offering protective benefits during this process. They do not need to be used simultaneously; applying both in the same day can be effective since the effects of the pack tend to be prolonged.

You can start with packs of 15, 30 to 60 minutes once a week and gradually increase to two or three times a week, eventually reaching daily use. It is possible to keep the thyroid pack on overnight, if desired. Everyone is different; one hour once a week may work for some individuals, while others may need more frequent use.

Oral Health

An Ayurvedic practice known as "oil pulling" helps maintain oral health. Traditionally done with sesame or coconut oil, the process involves swishing the oil in the mouth for 20 minutes and then spit it.

Recent research in periodontal medicine has shown that castor oil is highly effective in vivo (in the human body) when compared to traditional denture cleaners, particularly in breaking down biofilm[25] (the fuzzy feeling on teeth when you don't brush your teeth). This suggests that it can be used as part of oral hygiene to combat bacterial infections in the mouth, as this practice can help eliminate bad breath, nourish the gums, potentially whiten teeth, and balance the oral microbiome. Remarkably, these benefits can be achieved with just two minutes of castor oil pulling daily.

---

25   De Andrade, I. M., De Andrade, K. M., Pisani, M. X., Silva-Lovato, C. H., De Souza, R. F., & De Freitas Oliveira Paranhos, H. (2014). Trial of an Experimental Castor Oil Solution for Cleaning Dentures. *Brazilian Dental Journal,* 25(1), 43–47. | Badaró, M. M., Salles, M. M., Leite, V. M. F., De Arruda, C. N. F., De Cássia Oliveira, V., Nascimento, C. D., De Souza, R. F., De Freitas De Oliveira Paranhos, H., & Silva-Lovato, C. H. (2017). Clinical trial for evaluation of Ricinus communis and sodium hypochlorite as denture cleanser. *Journal of Applied Oral Science,* 25(3), 324–334. | Salles, M. M., Badaró, M. M., De Arruda, C. N. F., Leite, V. M. F., Da Silva, C. H. L., Watanabe, E., De Cássia Oliveira, V., & De Freitas Oliveira Paranhos, H. (2015). Antimicrobial activity of complete denture cleanser solutions based on sodium hypochlorite and Ricinus communis – a randomized clinical study. *Journal of Applied Oral Science,* 23(6), 637–642.

HOW TO USE CASTOR OIL FOR ORAL HYGIENE

A drop of castor oil applied to a cotton swab and dabbed on canker sores or gum infections can provide relief and promote healing.

For the practice of **oil pulling,** pour into your mouth about 1-2 teaspoons of castor oil. Swish the oil for about 2-5 minutes, ensuring the oil reaches all areas of your mouth, including under the tongue and between the teeth.

After swishing, spit the oil into a trash can (avoid spitting it into the sink or toilet as it can cause blockages). The oil should be milky white when you spit it out, indicating that it has mixed with saliva and captured toxins and bacteria. Thoroughly rinse your mouth with warm water to eliminate any residual oil. You can also use a natural mouthwash for a fresher feeling. You can brush your teeth before or after oil pulling.

Eye Health

In recent times, ophthalmologists have issued warnings against using **castor oil on eyelids** to treat vision problems, responding to claims circulating on social media platforms. Experts emphasize that castor oil can easily slip into the eye from the eyelid, potentially leading to irritation or other complications. They advise seeking professional medical advice for any vision-related issues.

Upon further investigation, their real concern is about the quality of the castor oil being used. Castor oils available on store shelves are not meant for eye use and may contain dyes, fragrances, preservatives, or other ingredients that can cause infection or irritation. Additionally, these oils may not be sterilized.

As we already know, there is no official scientific evidence to support the claim that rubbing castor oil on your eyelids enhances vision. However, many benefits are supported by extensive anecdotal evidence and the findings of interesting studies.

One crucial point to remember is that if you choose to use castor oil around your eyes, or on your eyelids, it is essential to use sterile, pharmaceutical-grade castor oil specifically formulated for eye use.

CASTOR OIL ON EYES

Legend has it that Cleopatra, the renowned Egyptian queen, used castor oil to enhance the brightness of the whites of her eyes. As the yellowing of the sclera, or its darkening, is a sign of aging, this use may represent one of the earliest practices to counteract aging. Historical references to castor oil for eye health date back to 1550 BC in a significant medical document called the Egyptian "Ebers Papyrus". Additionally, it is commonly used in India for corneal health and research has shown it is an effective remedy for dry eyes, particularly in Meibomian gland dysfunction[26].

Recent studies on rat lenses have shown that castor oil helps preserve glutathione, which is a crucial antioxidant of the eyes[27]. Glutathione is crucial for eye health because it protects the eyes from oxidative stress and damage caused by free radicals. It contributes to maintaining the clarity of the lens and it has demonstrated positive effects in preventing cataracts[28].

Additionally, glutathione supports the health of retinal cells, reducing the risk of age-related macular degeneration and other degenerative eye diseases. By detoxifying the eye tissues and supporting overall cellular health, glutathione plays a vital role in preserving vision and preventing various eye conditions.

Furthermore, A 2020 study demonstrated important improvements in ocular surface symptoms in patients with blepharitis after using castor oil. Improvements were noted in eyelid margin thickening, telangiectasia, cylindrical dandruff, and eyelash crusting[29].

Here are the effects that castor oil can have on the eyes, thanks to its unique chemical properties:

- **Moisturizing dry eyes**: it helps in lubricating the eyes, reducing dryness and irritation.
- **Anti-inflammatory properties**: it can reduce inflammation and soothe conditions like blepharitis.
- **Antimicrobial effects**: its antimicrobial properties can help prevent infections.
- **Healing conjunctivitis**: it can aid in the recovery from mild conjunctivitis due to its antimicrobial and anti-inflammatory effects.
- **Reducing redness and swelling**: the soothing properties can alleviate redness and swelling.

Interestingly, castor oil is a common ingredient included in some FDA-approved eye drops today.

26 Goto E1, Shimazaki J, Monden Y, Takano Y, Yagi Y, Shimmura S, Tsubota K. Low-concentration homogenized castor oil eye drops for noninflamed obstructive meibomian gland dysfunction. *Ophthalmology*. 2002 Nov;109(11):2030-5.

27 Holm, T., Brøgger-Jensen, M. R., Johnson, L., & Kessel, L. (2013b). Glutathione Preservation during Storage of Rat Lenses in Optisol-GS and Castor Oil. *PloS One*, 8(11), e79620.

28 Castor Oil & Age-Related Cataract – A Case for the Therapeutic Order. (2022, September 13). *Naturopathic Doctor News and Review*.

29 Muntz A, Sandford E, Claassen M, et al. Randomized trial of topical periocular castor oil treatment for blepharitis. *The Ocular Surface*. 2021;19:145-150.

The use of castor oil for health benefits has expanded into a popular trend: applying it to the belly button. This method, while not traditionally taught in naturopathic schools, has garnered significant attention on social media platforms.

Applying castor oil to the belly button is primarily used for acute daytime relief rather than the more extensive benefits of traditional castor oil packs. The process involves either pouring or rolling castor oil directly into the belly button and stimulating the area with a finger or roller.

The key benefit of this method is the stimulation of the vagus nerve, which induces a relaxation response, effectively acting as a rescue remedy for stress and anxiety. It provides immediate relief through the same vagus nerve stimulation that traditional packs offer, but it is more convenient for daytime use, helping to reduce symptoms such as gas, bloating, and overall digestive discomfort.

CHAPTER 4
CASTOR OIL FOR SKIN CARE

General Skin Health

Moisturizing and Emollient Properties

Castor oil is renowned for its exceptional moisturizing[30] and emollient properties. It is a versatile oil that can benefit various skin types, from dry to oily and even sensitive skin. Moreover, it does have antioxidants, specifically tocopherol and tocotrienols which are forms of vitamin E.

It is also important to mention that castor oil is non-comedogenic, making it a wonderful skin moisturizer that doesn't clog pores.

For **dry skin** castor oil is very beneficial because it is rich in ricinoleic acid, a fatty acid that has powerful humectant properties. This means it can attract and retain moisture in the skin, making it an excellent remedy for dry and flaky skin. It creates a protective barrier on the skin's surface, preventing the so called transepidermal water loss and keeping the skin hydrated for longer periods.

Although it might seem counterintuitive, castor oil can also benefit **oily skin**. The high concentration of ricinoleic acid can help balance the skin's natural oil production. By providing adequate moisture, it signals the skin to reduce the overproduction of sebum, which is often the cause of oily skin.

As castor oil has anti-inflammatory properties, it is suitable for **sensitive and irritated skin**. It can soothe redness, reduce inflammation, and provide a calming effect, making it a great option for those with conditions like eczema or rosacea. For sensitive skin, it's best to perform a patch test before full application.

Some people even use it under their eyes to reduce the appearance of dark circles, but here

---

30   Saraf, S., Sahu, S., Kaur, C. D., & Saraf, S. (2010). Comparative measurement of hydration effects of herbal moisturizers. *Pharmacognosy Research, 2*(3), 146.

are no scientific studies that back up claims that castor oil can treat under-eye circles, so it's mostly based on anecdotal evidence.

Castor oil is often used as a natural remedy to improve the health and appearance of nails. It is rich in fatty acids, which provide deep hydration to nails and cuticles, helping to prevent dryness and brittleness. Regular application of castor oil can help strengthen nails, reducing the likelihood of breakage and splitting, and promote growth thanks to its nutrients, including vitamin E and proteins. Additionally, castor oil has natural antifungal properties, which can help prevent and treat fungal infections on them.

APPLICATION TECHNIQUES

For **direct application** apply a few drops of castor oil directly to the skin and massage gently. This is particularly effective for dry and sensitive skin. As it can be very dense, it can also be mixed and diluted with other oils like jojoba oil or another emollient that is thinner in consistency, to facilitate application. For best results, use it at night to allow the oil to work while you sleep. Ensure the skin is clean before the treatment.

The oil cleansing method involves mixing castor oil with another carrier oil suitable for your skin type (e.g., jojoba oil for oily skin, coconut oil for dry skin). Massage the mixture into the skin for a few minutes, then remove it with a warm, damp cloth. Follow up with a gentle cleanser to remove any residual oil and impurities. This method helps maintain the skin's natural oil balance and removes makeup and dirt effectively.

You can also **improve your skincare products** by adding a few drops of castor oil to your regular moisturizer or serum. This can boost the hydrating properties of your skincare products without changing their consistency too much. Start with a small amount to avoid making the mixture too greasy. Adjust the ratio based on your skin's response.

For a **facial mask** combine castor oil with other natural ingredients like honey, aloe vera, or yogurt to create a hydrating and soothing facial mask. Apply it to your face and then leave it on for 15-20 minutes. Rinse off with warm water. Use this treatment once or twice a week to maintain skin hydration and suppleness.

Antimicrobial Effects

Castor oil has been recognized for its potent antimicrobial[31] properties, making it a valuable natural remedy for various skin infections and conditions.

---

31   Valera, M. C., Maekawa, L. E., De Oliveira, L. D., Jorge, A. O. C., Shygei, R., & Carvalho, C. a. T. (2013c). In vitro antimicrobial

Ricinoleic acid can inhibit the growth of several bacterial strains which are known to cause skin infections, boils, and other dermatological issues. It disrupts the bacterial cell membrane integrity, leading to cell lysis and death. This action makes castor oil effective in treating minor wounds, cuts, and abrasions by preventing **bacterial infections** and promoting healing.

Castor oil's antimicrobial and anti-inflammatory[32] properties can also help combat **acne**. It fights off acne-causing bacteria while reducing inflammation and redness associated with breakouts. Moreover, the antioxidants in it help slow down the oxidation of sebum, which is inflammatory and can worsen the condition of acne-prone skin.

Anything that is anti-inflammatory and moisturizing like castor oil can also aid in the clearance of **hyperpigmentation**, provided your skin is not exposed to unprotected sun or experiencing ongoing inflammation.

Castor oil can combat various fungal pathogens, such as candida albicans, which is responsible for yeast infections and **fungal dermatitis**. The oil's ability to penetrate deep into the skin enhances its effectiveness against these pathogens. Ricinoleic acid interferes with the cell wall synthesis of fungi, inhibiting their growth and reproduction. This makes castor oil a useful remedy for conditions like athlete's foot and ringworm.

RECOMMENDED TREATMENTS

Topical Application: for acne-prone skin, use castor oil as a spot treatment. Apply a small amount to affected areas using a cotton swab. It can also be incorporated into a nightly skincare routine by mixing it with non-comedogenic oils to prevent clogging pores.

For bacterial infections apply a small amount of castor oil directly to the affected area, still using a clean cotton swab, to treat minor cuts, wounds, and bacterial infections. Cover with a bandage if necessary to keep the area clean and protected. For fungal infections apply castor oil to the affected area twice daily, to treat conditions like athlete's foot or ringworm. Ensure the skin is dry and clean before application. Consistent use can help eliminate the fungal infection and prevent recurrence.

Castor Oil Packs: leave the pack on for at least an hour to enhance absorption and effectiveness. Castor oil packs can be particularly beneficial for larger areas of infection or inflamma-

---

activity of auxiliary chemical substances and natural extracts on Candida albicans and Enterococcus faecalis in root canals. *Journal of Applied Oral Science*, 21(2), 118–123.

32   Vieira, C., Evangelista, S., Cirillo, R., Lippi, A., Maggi, C. A., & Manzini, S. (2000b). Effect of ricinoleic acid in acute and subchronic experimental models of inflammation. *Mediators of Inflammation*, 9(5), 223–228 | Boddu, S. H., Alsaab, H., Umar, S., Bonam, S. P., Gupta, H., & Ahmed, S. (2015). Anti-inflammatory effects of a novel ricinoleic acid poloxamer gel system for transdermal delivery. *International Journal of Pharmaceutics*, 479(1), 207–211 | Yamamoto, Y., Harada, K., Kasuga, S., & Hosokawa, M. (2019). Phospholipase A2-Mediated preparation of phosphatidylcholine containing ricinoleic acid and its anti-inflammatory effect on murine macrophage-like RAW264.7 cells. *Biocatalysis and Agricultural Biotechnology*, 19, 101141

tion, such as fungal dermatitis or extensive bacterial skin infections. The heat helps increase blood flow to the area, promoting faster healing and more effective antimicrobial action.

For more in-depth information on how to use castor oil packs you can refer to Chapter 7.

Combination Treatments: combining castor oil with other antimicrobial essential oils, such as tea tree oil or lavender oil, can enhance its effectiveness. Mix a few drops of the essential oil with castor oil and apply to the affected area. This combination can provide broader-spectrum antimicrobial activity.

Wound Healing

Castor oil offers more than just moisturizing benefits for the skin, as it is also used as a natural remedy to promote wound healing.

A 2018 study published in *Polymers in Advanced Technology* found that castor oil may help reduce inflammation, alleviate pain, and support the healing process of wounds[33].

Research published in the *Journal of Wound, Ostomy, and Continence Nursing* in 2005 suggests that castor oil may aid in the recovery of wounds and pressure ulcers [34].

A 2016 study in *BMC Complementary and Alternative Medicine* found that castor oil has antibacterial properties effective against various bacteria, including *Staphylococcus aureus*, *Escherichia coli*, and *Pseudomonas aeruginosa*[35].

This suggests that castor oil may help reduce skin infections, lower the risk of staph infections, and support wound healing. Moreover, the increase of nitric oxide enhances blood flow to the affected area, supporting collagen synthesis, and modulating the activity of cells involved in tissue repair.

Castor oil can promote faster recovery from burns or abrasions, but it is not recommended for use on open wounds. Instead, it can be applied around the wound to enhance circulation and lymphatic drainage, which helps accelerate the healing process. It is also used post-surgery once the wound is healed to prevent the formation of tough scars and keloids, as these can obstruct the bioelectrical energy flow in the body.

Many women use castor oil packs postpartum on C-section scars, but it's crucial to wait until

33   Nada, A. A., Arul, M. R., Ramos, D. M., Kroneková, Z., Mosnáček, J., Rudraiah, S., & Kumbar, S. G. (2018). Bioactive polymeric formulations for wound healing. *Polymers for Advanced Technologies, 29*(6), 1815–1825.

34   Narayanan, S., Van Vleet, J., Strunk, B., Ross, R. N., & Gray, M. (2005). Comparison of Pressure Ulcer Treatments in Long-term Care Facilities. *Journal of Wound, Ostomy, and Continence Nursing/Journal of WOCN, 32*(3), 163–170

35   Al-Mamun, M. A., Akter, Z., Uddin, M. J., Ferdaus, K. M. K. B., Hoque, K. M. F., Ferdousi, Z., & Reza, M. A. (2016). Characterization and evaluation of antibacterial and antiproliferative activities of crude protein extracts isolated from the seed of Ricinus communis in Bangladesh. *BMC Complementary and Alternative Medicine, 16*(1)

the incision has fully healed. Once the stitches are out and a scar has formed, applying a castor oil pelvic pack can promote better scar formation and prevent keloids, which are caused by excessive inflammation. This practice helps the body recover post-pregnancy by improving circulation and lymphatic drainage. Additionally, using pelvic packs can benefit breastfeeding, as it supports ovarian function, which in turn affects milk production. This holistic approach helps reset the body's systems postpartum.

Reducing Scarring and Stretch Marks

We have substantial anecdotal evidence of positive experiences using castor oil to reduce scarring. Users have reported noticeable fading of post-surgery scars within a few months of regular application. The skin around the scars became smoother, and the redness reduced significantly. Also people with acne scars, or even stretch marks, have experienced significant lightening and improvement in skin texture. Consistent application of castor oil has resulted in smoother and clearer skin over time.

APPLICATION GUIDE

Begin by thoroughly cleaning the area you wish to treat with a gentle cleanser and warm water and pat the area dry with a soft towel. Pour a small amount of castor oil into your palm or onto a clean cotton ball, and gently massage the oil into the affected area using circular motions. Ensure that the oil is evenly distributed and covers the entire scar area. Place a clean cloth or bandage over the treated area, as this helps to keep the oil in place and allows it to penetrate deeper into the skin. For larger areas, you may use a piece of plastic wrap to prevent the oil from transferring to your clothing.

For optimal results, leave the castor oil on for at least an hour. If possible, leave it on overnight. This extended exposure allows the oil's properties to work more effectively. After the desired time has passed, if you want you can rinse off the castor oil with warm water and a mild soap and then apply a light moisturizer if needed.

Consistency is key to seeing results. Repeat this process at least daily and for several weeks to observe significant improvements.

Smoothing Wrinkles and Fine Lines

Castor oil has garnered significant attention in the realm of skincare due to its potent anti-aging properties. One of the primary benefits of castor oil is its ability to smooth wrinkles and fine lines. When applied topically, castor oil penetrates deep into the skin layers, providing intense hydration. This deep moisturizing effect helps to plump up the skin, reducing the appearance of fine lines and wrinkles.

Moreover, vitamin E helps reduce oxidation of lipids on the top layers your skin (due to environmental conditions and pollution), which triggers an inflammatory cascade that can contribute to premature skin aging and the formation of wrinkles. Castor oil can potentially slow or reduce the effects of premature skin aging.

APPLICATION TECHNIQUES

Apply a few drops of castor oil directly to the face, focusing on areas with fine lines and wrinkles. Gently massage the oil into the skin using circular motions to enhance absorption. You can even soak a piece of cloth in castor oil and place it over the face for 15-20 minutes, for prolonged contact with the skin and maximized the anti-aging benefits. For enhanced benefits, mix castor oil with other anti-aging oils like argan oil or rosehip oil. This combination provides a broader spectrum of nutrients that nourish the skin.

Today, castor oil is frequently found in eye creams. The skin around the eyes is extremely fragile and sensitive, so it is important to be cautious about the products we use in this area. Castor oil, when free of dyes, fragrances, or preservatives, is entirely safe for application around and in the eyes, making it a gentle and effective choice for eye care.

Promoting Skin Elasticity

In addition to smoothing wrinkles, castor oil is highly effective in promoting skin elasticity. This property is crucial for maintaining a firm and toned complexion. The unique composition of castor oil, rich in fatty acids, vitamins, and minerals, nourishes the skin and enhances its elasticity.

Fatty acids in castor oil, such as ricinoleic acid, oleic acid, and linoleic acid, play a vital role in maintaining the skin's barrier function. They prevent water loss, ensuring the skin remains hydrated and supple. Well-hydrated skin is more elastic and resilient, reducing the likelihood of sagging and the formation of new wrinkles.

APPLICATION TECHNIQUES

As an **overnight treatment**, apply a thin layer of castor oil to the face and neck before bed. Leave it on overnight to let the skin fully absorb the nutrients. In the morning, wash it off with a gentle cleanser.

You can also incorporate castor oil into your **facial massage routine**. Regular massage with castor oil enhances blood circulation, promoting the delivery of nutrients and oxygen to the skin cells. This process supports the skin's natural repair mechanisms, improving elasticity.

Hyaluronic acid is another powerful ingredient known for its hydrating properties. When combined with castor oil, it creates a potent anti-aging treatment. Apply hyaluronic acid serum to the face, followed by a layer of castor oil to lock in moisture and enhance elasticity.

CHAPTER 5
CASTOR OIL FOR HAIR CARE

Hair Growth and Health

The field of hair growth science has garnered significant attention over the years, leading to a growing body of knowledge. Research has extensively explored the various signaling molecules the body utilizes to regulate the hair growth cycle, with prostaglandins being a key player.

As discussed in the second chapter of this book, prostaglandins are a diverse group of agents involved in numerous physiological processes. Notably, scientists have discovered their role in hair growth and darkening. The study of eyelash hair growth for cosmetic purposes is particularly prominent. Bimatoprost, a prostaglandin analogue, has received FDA approval for treating hypotrichosis of the eyelashes (insufficient or inadequate eyelashes). Bimatoprost has demonstrated its ability to stimulate eyelash growth in vivo, human scalp hair growth in vitro, and mouse pelage hair growth in vivo[36].

Furthermore, research on hair follicles, beginning in 2008, revealed that the expression of prostaglandin receptors increases before and during the growth phase of the hair cycle. Prostaglandin E2 (PGE2) plays a crucial role in the anagen phase (growth phase) of the hair cycle, promoting the growth of thicker and healthier hair. These findings suggest that using a prostaglandin analogue could yield promising results for hair growth enhancement[37].

The chemical structure of ricinoleic acid, found in castor oil, is similar to prostaglandins (see Chapter 2 for more details). This similarity suggests that ricinoleic acid could mimic prostaglandin activity, potentially impacting hair growth when it penetrates the hair follicle.

Early animal studies provide compelling evidence to further investigate castor oil as a treat-

---

36   Khidhir, K. G., Woodward, D. F., Farjo, N. P., Farjo, B. K., Tang, E. S., Wang, J. W., Picksley, S. M., & Randall, V. A. (2012). The prostamide-related glaucoma therapy, bimatoprost, offers a novel approach for treating scalp alopecias. *the FASEB Journal*, 27(2), 557–567.

37   Jiang, S., Hao, Z., Qi, W., Wang, Z., Zhou, M., & Guo, N. (2023). The efficacy of topical prostaglandin analogs for hair loss: A systematic review and meta-analysis. *Frontiers in Medicine*, 10.

ment for hair loss and thinning. One particular study demonstrated that when castor oil was mixed with lotion and applied topically, it significantly enhanced hair growth[38].

In certain instances, hair loss results from inflammation of the hair follicles. Applying castor oil to the scalp can alleviate follicle inflammation and enhance blood flow to the area through nitric oxide[39]. Additionally, castor oil delivers growth-promoting nutrients such as omega fatty acids and vitamin E.

What we know is that castor oil has long been celebrated for its beneficial effects on hair growth and health. Many people report that using castor oil on their scalp improves hair growth or reverses hair loss. Additionally, castor oil is popular as a natural lash and brow serum, promoting lash and brow growth and enhancement.

Stimulating Hair Follicles

The ability of castor oil to stimulate hair follicles is primarily attributed to its ability to promote blood circulation to the scalp[40]. Improved blood circulation guarantees that the hair follicles receive adequate oxygen and nutrients, which are crucial for hair growth.

In addition to promoting blood flow, castor oil possesses anti-inflammatory properties. Inflammation of the scalp can impede hair growth by damaging hair follicles and inhibiting their ability to function properly. The anti-inflammatory effects of ricinoleic acid help soothe the scalp and create a healthy environment for hair follicles to thrive.

APPLICATION TECHNIQUES

Gently massage warm castor oil into the **scalp** using circular motions. This stimulates blood circulation and helps the oil penetrate deeply into the hair follicles. Leave the oil on for at least 1 hour or overnight for best results. You can wear a shower cap, or if you use it overnight cover your pillow with an old towel. Wash it out with a mild shampoo. You can repeat the treatment once a week.

On **eyebrows** use a clean mascara wand or brow brush for easier application. If you don't have either, a clean Q-tip will suffice. Start by washing your face with a gentle cleanser and patting it dry. Dip the brush into a small bowl containing a bit of castor oil, allowing any excess

---

38   Kesika, P., Sivamaruthi, B. S., Thangaleela, S., Bharathi, M., & Chaiyasut, C. (2023). Role and Mechanisms of Phytochemicals in Hair Growth and Health. *Pharmaceuticals*, *16*(2), 206.

39   Mascolo N1, Izzo AA, Autore G, Barbato F, Capasso F. Nitric oxide and castor oil-induced diarrhea. *Journal of Pharmacology and Experimental Therapeutics*. 1994 Jan;268(1):291-5.

40   Rusu M., Csedo C., Marcus G., Lupuliasa D. Preclinical study on the hair growth and regeneration of external use lotions containing castor oil (*Ricini oleum*) in rabbits. Farmacia. 2008;56:507–512

to drip off. Gently brush each eyebrow to coat the hairs with a thin layer of oil, being careful to avoid any dripping into your eyes. Make sure to get to the roots. The required amount will vary depending on the thickness of your eyebrows; thinner brows need less oil. Depending on your routine, you can leave the castor oil on for a few hours or overnight. When it's time to remove the oil, wash your face as usual. If irritation occurs, rinse off the oil immediately. In case of contact with eyes, flush with clean water.

For **eyelashes** follow the same steps as for eyebrows, ensuring your mascara wand is clean. Apply the oil carefully to your top and bottom lashes, similar to how you would apply mascara, avoiding contact with your eyes but trying to get to the roots. The oil can be applied for a few hours or left on overnight. Before applying any cosmetics, make sure to wash off the oil thoroughly using warm water and a gentle cleanser.

Reducing Hair Breakage and Split Ends

Hair breakage and split ends are common issues that can lead to hair appearing thin and unhealthy. Castor oil's high viscosity helps it form a protective coating on the hair shaft, which can prevent damage from external factors such as pollution, heat styling, and chemical treatments. This protective barrier helps to maintain the structural integrity of the hair and reduces the likelihood of breakage and split ends.

Moreover, castor oil is an excellent moisturizer due to its high content of fatty acids. These fatty acids penetrate deeply into the hair shaft, providing much-needed hydration to dry and brittle hair. Well-moisturized hair is less prone to breakage and split ends, as it is more flexible and resilient.

The emollient properties of castor oil also help to smooth the hair cuticle, the outermost layer of the hair shaft. When the cuticle is smooth, the hair strands lie flat, resulting in less friction and tangling. This not only reduces breakage but also gives the hair a shinier and healthier appearance.

APPLICATION TECHNIQUES

Combine castor oil with other beneficial oils, such as coconut oil or olive oil (optional), to create a nourishing **hair mask** as a pre-shampoo treatment. Apply the mixture to the hair and scalp, focusing on the ends. Cover your hair with a shower cap and leave the mask on for 1-2 hours before washing it out.

As a **split end treatment**, apply a small amount of castor oil to the ends of your hair as a leave-in conditioner to prevent breakage. This can be done daily or as needed to keep the ends hydrated and healthy.

Scalp Treatments with Castor Oil

Scalp health is an essential aspect of overall hair health, and issues like dandruff and dry scalp can significantly impact both appearance and comfort.

Addressing Dandruff and Dry Scalp

Dandruff is characterized by flaky skin on the scalp, often accompanied by itching and irritation. It can be caused by several factors, including fungal infections, dry skin, sensitivity to hair products, and seborrheic dermatitis. Dry scalp, on the other hand, occurs when the scalp lacks sufficient moisture, leading to itching, flaking, and irritation. Both conditions can be distressing and challenging to manage.

Castor oil can be an effective treatment for both dandruff and dry scalp due to its moisturizing and emollient properties.

APPLICATION TECHNIQUES

Using circular motions, gently massage castor oil into the scalp. Leave the oil on for at least 30 minutes or overnight for best results, wash it out with a mild shampoo and repeat the treatment as often as needed.

When applied to the scalp, castor oil provides deep hydration, replenishing the moisture levels and helping to soothe and calm dry, irritated skin. This hydration helps to reduce flaking and itching associated with dry scalp and dandruff. Regular application of castor oil can improve overall scalp health by creating a healthier environment for hair growth. The oil forms a protective barrier, preventing moisture loss and maintaining a balanced, hydrated state.

Antifungal and Antibacterial Properties

The properties of castor oil play a crucial role in addressing dandruff, which is often caused by fungal infections such as Malassezia. Ricinoleic acid with its potent antifungal properties helps to inhibit the growth of Malassezia and other fungal species that contribute to dandruff, as nitric oxide is a strong anti-yeast and anti-fungal agent[41].

Moreover, the oil's ability to fight off harmful bacteria ensures that the scalp remains clean and free from infections, promoting a healthier environment for hair growth.

---

41   Mascolo N1, Izzo AA, Autore G, Barbato F, Capasso F. Nitric oxide and castor oil-induced diarrhea. *Journal of Pharmacology and Experimental Therapeutics.* 1994 Jan;268(1):291-5.

APPLICATION TECHNIQUES

Warm a small amount of castor oil in your hands and **massage** it directly into the scalp. Focus on areas with the most flaking or irritation. Leave the oil on for at least 30 minutes, or overnight for deeper hydration, before washing it out with a mild shampoo.

Combine castor oil with other beneficial ingredients, such as coconut oil or aloe vera gel, to create a **hydrating scalp mask**. Apply the mask to the scalp, leave it on for 30-60 minutes, and then rinse thoroughly. This combination can provide enhanced moisturizing and soothing effects.

For best results, incorporate castor oil treatments into your **regular hair care routine**. Using castor oil 1-2 times a week can help maintain scalp health and prevent the recurrence of dandruff and dryness.

CHAPTER 6
FEMALE WELLNESS AND CASTOR OIL

Introduction

In this transformative chapter we will delve into the myriad benefits of castor oil for female wellness. From addressing hormonal imbalances to easing menstrual discomfort, this natural remedy has found a special place in women's health care.

Hormone Cycling

First, let's gain a better understanding of hormone cycling in women. This comprehensive overview will help us see how castor oil can be beneficial from various perspectives.

Hormone cycling is a natural and intricate process that governs the female reproductive system, involving a delicate interplay between the hypothalamus, pituitary gland, and ovaries, which regulate the menstrual cycle through a series of hormonal signals.

The cycle is divided into two main phases:

Follicular Phase (Day 1 to Ovulation)

The hypothalamus releases a hormone (GnRH), which prompts the pituitary gland to secrete follicle-stimulating hormone (FSH). FSH stimulates the ovaries to produce estrogen and facilitate the growth of follicles, one of which will mature into an egg. As estrogen levels rise, they prepare the uterine lining for potential implantation and signal the pituitary to release luteinizing hormone (LH), which triggers ovulation.

During the follicular phase the body is preparing for potential implantation by cleaning up and detoxifying.

Luteal Phase (Post-Ovulation to Day 28)

Post-ovulation, in the luteal phase, the ruptured follicle transforms into the corpus luteum, which secretes progesterone to sustain the uterine lining and support early pregnancy if fertilization occurs. If pregnancy does not occur, progesterone levels fall, leading to menstruation and the start of a new cycle.

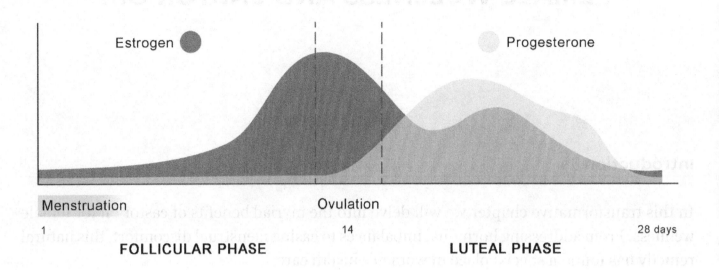

Women's hormones are a complex system that maintains a delicate balance, influenced by factors like diet, exercise, sleep, stress levels, and environmental toxins. Disruptions in any of these areas can lead to hormonal imbalances. Even a slight imbalance can cause various health issues, such as irregular periods, acne, PCOS, thyroid disorders, and chronic fatigue.

The prevalence of these conditions indicates that many women are affected by disruptions in their hormonal balance, making it a common health issue that requires attention and management.

Supporting Hormonal Balance

An imbalance in hormone levels can frequently lead to irregular periods, weight fluctuations, hair loss, and a variety of other health problems.

Hormone cycling with castor oil is a method used to align the application of castor oil packs with the phases of a woman's menstrual cycle. The aim is to support the body's natural rhythms and, in turn, to support hormonal balance.

Here's how castor oil packs help maintain a balanced hormonal environment.

The **follicular phase**, from bleeding to ovulation, is the optimal time for detoxification and cleansing because the body's energy is concentrated in the liver. The liver breaks down excess hormones, particularly estrogen, thus preventing estrogen dominance—a common cause of menstrual irregularities, PMS (premenstrual syndrome), and conditions such as polycystic ovary syndrome (PCOS). During this phase, applying **castor oil packs over the liver** significantly regulates hormonal cycling by enhancing the body's natural detoxification processes. This promotes a more efficient breakdown of excess estrogen and improves the hormonal environment for follicle development.

In the luteal phase, from ovulation to bleeding, all the focus and the energy of the female body shifts into the pelvic region, as it's all about nourishment of the uterus in preparation for implantation. Applying castor oil packs to the pelvic region during this phase promotes uterine health and hormonal balance. **Castor oil packs to the pelvic area** can enhance circulation and lymphatic drainage, reducing pelvic congestion and supporting the health of the corpus luteum, thereby stabilizing progesterone levels. This helps to maintain the uterine lining and reduces the likelihood of PMS symptoms and irregular cycles.

CASTOR OIL PACKS BENEFITS

Here are some ways castor oil packs support hormonal balance in women, based on how ricinoleic acid acts:

- **Improving Liver Function**: ricinoleic acid in castor oil aids the liver in detoxifying the body. This process helps prevent estrogen dominance, which can lead to hormonal imbalances.
- **Reducing Inflammation**: ricinoleic acid has potent anti-inflammatory properties that help reduce inflammation in the body. Inflammation can interfere with hormone production and regulation, so minimizing it is crucial for maintaining hormonal balance.
- **Enhancing Circulation**: using castor oil packs improves blood flow to reproductive organs, ensuring they receive adequate nutrients and oxygen. Enhanced circulation supports the optimal function of these organs, which is vital for hormone production and regulation.
- **Stimulating Prostaglandin Production**: ricinoleic acid can mimic the action of prostaglandins, which are compounds involved in regulating various bodily functions, including the menstrual cycle. By stimulating prostaglandin production, castor oil packs help regulate hormones and menstrual cycles.
- **Supporting Lymphatic System**: castor oil packs enhance lymphatic drainage, which helps remove toxins and waste products from the body. An efficient lymphatic system is crucial for maintaining hormonal balance as it prevents the buildup of toxins that can disrupt endocrine function.
- **Reducing Cystic Formations**: castor oil packs can also help reduce cysts in various body areas, including ovarian cysts, fibroids, and fibrocystic breasts, providing a holistic approach to managing systemic inflammation and hormonal imbalances.

As a general guideline, it typically takes about three months to notice significant changes in your body related to balanced hormones. However, you may observe some immediate improvements, such as better sleep, enhanced bowel movements, and reduced stress. These early changes occur as your hormones begin to align properly.

For more in-depth information on how to use castor oil packs you can refer to Chapter 7.

Castor Oil and the Moon

Anthropological evidence suggests that women traditionally aligned their menstrual cycles with lunar phases. Modern research also supports this connection, making this insight useful for women experiencing irregular or ceased menstrual cycles.

Studies suggest that the new moon often coincides with the onset of menstruation, meaning that for many women, the new moon phase aligns with the start of their menstrual cycle. Consequently, the ovulatory phase, which occurs approximately midway through the cycle, would coincide with the full moon. This lunar influence on menstrual cycles implies a potential synchronization where menstrual onset is linked to the new moon, and ovulation aligns with the full moon.

In summary, the **follicular phase** starts from the **new moon** and continues until the full moon, while the **luteal phase** begins with the **full moon** and lasts until the new moon, as illustrated in the following table.

MENSTRUAL CYCLE PHASE	CORRESPONDING MOON PHASE		DESCRIPTION
Menstrual phase		New Moon (the moon is entirely in shadow, with a dark surface)	Menstruation typically starts, reflecting new beginnings and cleansing.
Follicular Phase		Waxing Crescent to First Quarter	Body prepares for ovulation, developing follicles, and building up estrogen levels.
Ovulatory Phase		Full Moon (the entire face of the moon is illuminated)	Ovulation occurs, optimal fertility time, peak of estrogen levels.
Luteal Phase		Waning Gibbous to Last Quarter	After ovulation, the body prepares for potential pregnancy, progesterone levels rise.
Pre-Menstrual Phase		Waning Crescent	If no pregnancy, hormone levels drop, leading to menstruation and the cycle restarts.

APPLICATION TECHNIQUES

As a result, here's how castor oil packs should be used to enhance hormonal balance based on the moon cycles:

- start the **liver pack on the new moon** and continue until the full moon, as this phase corresponds to the follicular phase
- switch to the **pelvic pack from the full moon** until the new moon, as the luteal phase takes place.

Enhancing Fertility

For women seeking to enhance their fertility, castor oil offers several benefits as it supports hormonal balance and reproductive health by improving circulation, reducing inflammation, and promoting detoxification.

If your menstrual cycle is regular, you can use the follicular and luteal phases to apply castor oil packs first on the liver and then on the pelvic area. To achieve overall hormonal balance, consider taking care of your thyroid as well (a dedicated paragraph follows this chapter). As we have learned, our body functions as a system, with all organs playing important roles.

For irregular cycles, you can follow the moon phases and adhere to the same routine.

Use a castor oil pack every 2-4 days for at least one hour to enhance fertility, noting that more frequent use yields better results. If you have endometriosis, fibroids, or ovarian cysts, you can use the pack every day or every other day, keeping it on overnight for optimal results.

For more in-depth information on how to use castor oil packs you can refer to Chapter 7.

Alleviating Discomfort

Menstrual cramps and discomfort are pervasive issues that a significant number of women experience monthly. These symptoms, often manifesting as throbbing or cramping pains in the lower abdomen, can vary in intensity from mild to severe, sometimes interfering with daily activities.

The discomfort is typically caused by the contraction of the uterine muscles as they expel the uterine lining. This natural process can lead to associated symptoms such as bloating, back pain, and headaches. Menstrual pain during bleeding or ovulation indicates stagnation. Castor oil penetrates deeply, soothes the nervous system, breaks up stagnation, and restores proper flow.

Castor oil is also highly beneficial for certain conditions, especially if you have blockages or masses such as blocked tubes, fibroids, endometriosis, cysts, or polyps. It penetrates deeply into the body, gently softening and breaking down scar tissue, adhesions, and other abnormalities. This process aids in the gradual removal of these issues from the body, alleviating inflammation and pain.

Place a castor oil pack on the lower abdomen during your menstrual cycle. If you prefer, you can place something warm on top of it, like a heating pad or warm compress Use it for one hour or overnight for best results.

This practice can significantly reduce menstrual cramps and discomfort. Castor oil packs promote circulation, increasing blood flow to the pelvic area, which helps to ease cramps and reduce pain. Additionally, the warming effect of castor oil packs relaxes the uterine muscles, further reducing the intensity of menstrual cramps.

Perimenopause / Menopause / Seeking a Child-Free Life

Perimenopause is the transitional phase before menopause, marked by varying hormone levels, especially estrogen and progesterone. Women may encounter hot flashes, night sweats, mood swings, irregular periods, and sleep disturbances.

Menopause marks the end of menstrual cycles, typically confirmed after 12 consecutive months without a period. This stage brings about a more stable but lower level of estrogen and progesterone, often resulting in symptoms like vaginal dryness, reduced libido, bone density loss, and increased risk of cardiovascular issues.

Regular use of castor oil packs during perimenopause and menopause can lead to long-term benefits, including reduced severity of menopausal symptoms, better overall hormonal health, and a smoother transition through these stages. Women who maintain this practice may experience fewer health issues related to hormonal imbalance and enjoy better quality of life.

APPLICATION TECHNIQUES

The protocol for using castor oil packs in perimenopause and menopause follows an opposite cycle, which is also ideal for **women who do not want to get pregnant**. This approach maintains the benefits of castor oil pack treatment while catering to different reproductive goals and relies on the moon phases:

- Start the **liver pack** on the **full moon** and continue until the new moon.
- when the **new moon** arrives, switch the pack to your **pelvic area** and continue using it until the full moon.

Here are the significant benefits that castor oil packs can provide in these cases:

1. Hormonal balance and symptom relief: castor oil packs detoxify and reduce inflammation, and this is crucial during perimenopause and menopause when hormone levels are in flux. Regular use of castor oil packs can help alleviate common symptoms such as hot flashes, night sweats, and mood swings by stabilizing hormone levels and enhancing liver function, which is essential for hormone metabolism.

2. Stress reduction and improved sleep: stress and poor sleep are common issues during perimenopause and menopause. Castor oil packs can induce a state of relaxation, helping to shift the body into a parasympathetic state, which is crucial for healing and recovery. This relaxed state can improve sleep quality, reduce anxiety, and help manage mood swings, making it easier for women to cope with the emotional challenges of hormonal changes.

3. Enhanced detoxification: the liver plays a vital role in processing and eliminating hormones from the body. Castor oil can be particularly beneficial during perimenopause and menopause when the liver is tasked with managing the hormonal fluctuations. A healthy liver can better regulate hormone levels, reducing the severity and frequency of symptoms.

4. Anti-inflammatory and antioxidant benefits: castor oil is rich in antioxidants like vitamin E and has natural anti-inflammatory properties. These attributes can help reduce inflammation in the body, which is often heightened during perimenopause and menopause, alleviating joint pain, improving skin health, and supporting overall well-being.

5. Support for bone health: maintaining bone density is a significant concern during menopause due to the drop in estrogen levels, which can lead to osteoporosis. While castor oil packs are not a direct treatment for bone density, their ability to support overall hormonal balance and reduce inflammation can indirectly benefit bone health. A well-functioning liver and balanced hormones contribute to better calcium metabolism and bone strength.

The Role of Thyroid

The thyroid gland significantly impacts women's reproductive health, with thyroid hormones playing an important role in maintaining regular menstrual cycles and fertility.

Hypothyroidism, characterized by low thyroid hormone levels, can disrupt the menstrual cycle, causing heavy or prolonged menstrual bleeding, or infrequent menstruation. It can also interfere with ovulation, leading to difficulties in conceiving. It may also increase the risk of miscarriage in early pregnancy.

Conversely, **hyperthyroidism**, marked by excessive thyroid hormone production, can result in lighter or absent menstrual periods, impacting fertility.

Proper thyroid function ensures balanced hormone levels, essential for regular ovulation, healthy menstrual cycles, and overall reproductive health.

HOW CASTOR OIL PACKS HELP

When the thyroid pack is incorporated into a comprehensive practice to balance female hormones using castor oil packs, its benefits become even more significant.

When trying to achieve hormonal balance, even more importantly in the presence of thyroid issues, thyroid packs should be incorporated into the complete process that comprehends liver and pelvic packs during the particular phases of the menstrual cycle.

During the **follicular phase** (from menstruation to ovulation) the liver breaks down excess hormones, so applying **castor oil packs over the liver** significantly helps by enhancing the body's natural detoxification processes. But, as we have learned in the Chapter 3, when using castor oil packs on liver we should protect the thyroid at the same time, especially in the presence of thyroid issues. So in this phase we should apply a **castor oil pack to the thyroid** too to reduce inflammation and potential damage. Apply the castor oil pack for one hour a day, and the liver pack for at least an hour and ideally overnight.

In the **luteal phase** (from ovulation to menstruation), applying **castor oil packs to the pelvic region** promotes uterine health and hormonal balance. Pairing this with a **breast castor oil pack** is beneficial as the focus is not on detoxing, but on nourishing and breaking down blockages in the ovaries, uterus, and breasts, alleviating issues such as ovarian health impacts, uterine dysfunction, and breast tenderness. Castor oil packs on the breast can also help reduce fibrotic tissue and cysts. Apply the packs on the pelvic area and on the breast for at least one hour each, or ideally overnight.

Here's an easy trick to remember how application changes: the liver pack drops down to the pelvic pack, and the thyroid pack drops down to the breast pack.

For women experiencing irregular or ceased menstrual cycles the whole method can be repeated following the moon cycle, as we have learned, in order to regulate hormone balance effectively.

Pregnancy and Post-Partum

Castor oil can stimulate uterine contractions, posing a risk of preterm labor; therefore, pregnant women must avoid using it both internally and externally as a pack.

However, postpartum and while breastfeeding, castor oil packs can be beneficial.

When applied to the pelvic region, they may help reset organs and improve milk production by supporting ovarian health. It is recommended to avoid liver packs during breastfeeding to prevent active liver movement because stimulating the liver can lead to the release of stored toxins into the bloodstream, and these toxins might be transferred to the breast milk. By focusing on the pelvic pack instead, the organs can gradually return to their proper positions post-birth without the additional challenge of detoxification, ensuring a safer environment for both mother and baby during the breastfeeding period.

After breastfeeding, women can cycle again between liver and pelvic packs to support hormonal balance.

IUDs - Intrauterine Devices

There is some hearsay suggesting that you can't use a castor oil pack if you have an IUD, but this isn't true. In many Naturopathic Doctors' practice, thousands of patients use IUDs, particularly copper IUDs, without any issues. They monitored their mineral levels closely and never encountered problems with IUDs coming out due to castor oil packs. This method of birth control remained effective and safe even with the use of castor oil packs.

CHAPTER 7
CASTOR OIL PACKS

Introduction

Although historical use of castor oil dates back to ancient civilizations (ancient Egyptians around 1550 BC), its use in packs or wraps is often attributed to the early 20th century and the work of Edgar Cayce, an American mystic and medical clairvoyant. Cayce promoted the use of castor oil packs for a variety of health issues. His holistic approach and detailed readings on the use of castor oil packs helped popularize this method in modern alternative and complementary medicine practices. The resurgence of castor oil packs in traditional medicine has been championed by Naturopathic Doctors, Holistic Practitioners, Nutritionists, and health food stores. Many professionals make it their first recommendation to patients and clients, highlighting the packs' benefits in promoting health and wellness.

Castor oil packs involve the application of castor oil-soaked cloths to the skin, typically over specific areas of the body, to harness the anti-inflammatory, detoxifying, and lymphatic-stimulating properties of castor oil. They are recommended for various conditions including irritable bowel syndrome (IBS), inflammatory bowel diseases (IBD) like Crohn's and colitis, constipation, GERD (Gastroesophageal reflux disease), stress, anxiety, general detoxification, a weakened immune system, gastritis, hormonal imbalances, infertility, and even cancer. Essentially, they are beneficial for a wide range of health issues, except during pregnancy.

The Mechanism of Castor Oil Packs

When discussing the effectiveness of castor oil packs, it's essential to understand the unique mechanism that differentiates them from merely applying castor oil to the skin.

The key lies in the combination of the castor oil, the organic cotton flannel of the pack, and the sustained compression they provide. This synergistic approach is what makes castor oil packs a potent therapeutic tool.

The pack is a critical component of the treatment. When people simply rub castor oil on their skin and cover it with a T-shirt, they miss out on the therapeutic benefits provided by the compression, which accounts for 50% of the treatment's effectiveness. The covering and the pressure exerted by the soft organic cotton flannel, especially one that is delicate and fuzzy like sherpa, are what makes the difference and triggers a relaxation response via somatic-visceral reflexes.

Penetration

To achieve systemic effects, castor oil must penetrate into the dermis, which lies beneath the stratum corneum and three other epidermal layers: granular, spinous, and basal. The dermis is rich in blood vessels and lymphatic connections, facilitating the distribution of castor oil throughout the body.

Mechanical support is necessary to help the oil penetrate these layers, ensuring maximum absorption and efficacy. Modern transdermal therapy guidelines say that: "The major products currently marketed for transdermal absorption are the transdermal therapeutic systems (TTS), popularly known as patches. The functional parts of a patch, proceeding from the visible surface inward to the surface apposed to the skin, are: 1. An impermeable backing; 2. A reservoir holding the active ingredient…; 3. An adhesive to hold the patch in place on the skin; 4. A protective cover that is peeled away before applying the patch" [(Scheindlin, S. (2004b). *Transdermal Drug Delivery: PAST, PRESENT, FUTURE.* Molecular Interventions, 4(6), 308–312.)].

For castor oil packs, the oil is either poured onto layers of organic cotton flannel, then covered with a material to hold the pack in place, such as plastic wrap, or it is applied to the internal surface of modern pre-made packs, which have an impermeable backing. These contemporary packs come with incorporated straps to ensure they stay securely in place.

The molecular composition of the drug also plays its important role: "Although the stratum corneum is an efficient barrier, some chemical substances are able to penetrate it and to reach the underlying tissues and blood vessels. These "successful" substances are characterized by low molecular weight (≤500 Da)" [(Scheindlin, S. (2004b). *Transdermal Drug Delivery: PAST, PRESENT, FUTURE.* Molecular Interventions, 4(6), 308–312.)].

As we have learned, ricinoleic acid has a molecular weight of approximately 298.46 Daltons, so it is able to permeate through the lower layer of the epidermis and reach the areas where blood and lymphatic vessels reside.

Packs apply mechanical pressure, create tension, and retain natural body heat in the area, which opens pores and enables the oil to penetrate the skin through the roots of hair follicles. Without a pack, castor oil would not go as deeply and would mainly function as a skin moisturizer, limiting its full range of benefits.

Body's Response

The packs should be made with specific softness and must cover certain dermatomes (areas of skin receiving sensory innervation) to be effective and enhance the body's neurological response.

The specific softness and gentle pressure from the pack stimulates specific sensory receptors in the skin: **C-tactile afferent nerves** are specialized sensory fibers that respond to gentle, slow, and caressing touch; **Merkel's discs** are mechanoreceptors that detect sustained pressure and texture. Both are crucial in sending signals to the brain that are interpreted as soothing and calming.

The stimulation creates a cascade of neurological responses, and play a crucial role in activating the **vagus nerve**, which is a major component of the parasympathetic nervous system. Stimulating the vagus nerve triggers a relaxation response, shifting the body into a "rest and digest" mode.

This process is similar to the satisfaction felt after consuming a fatty meal, and involves the release of several key neurotransmitters such as **oxytocin** and **dopamine**. Oxytocin, often referred to as the "love hormone," fosters a sense of well-being and bonding, while dopamine is crucial for the reward and pleasure centers of the brain, contributing to feelings of happiness and satisfaction.

This shift to the relaxed state lowers heart rate and blood pressure, reduces stress levels, and promotes overall healing. Enhanced vagal tone allows the body to focus on processes like digestion, detoxification, immune function and tissue repair.

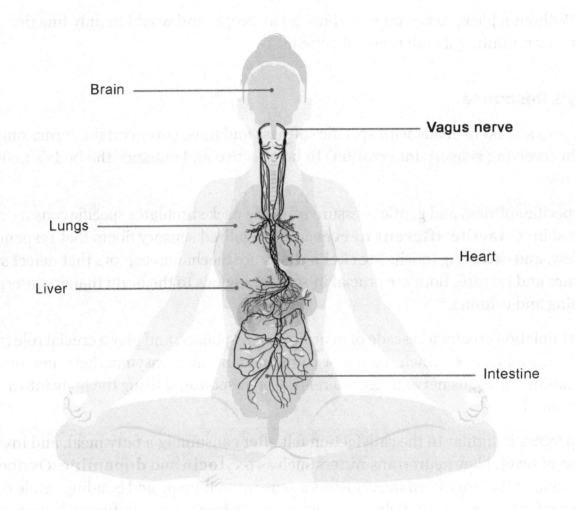

Brain

Vagus nerve

Lungs

Heart

Liver

Intestine

The **vagus nerve** is a cranial nerve involved in the parasympathetic regulation of the heart, lungs, and digestive tract. It consists of two nerves—the left and right vagus nerves—each containing approximately 100,000 fibers, but they are commonly referred to together as one subsystem. The vagus was also historically called the **pneumogastric nerve** [*Vagus nerve*. (2024, June 8). Wikipedia.]

Creating and Applying Castor Oil Packs

Castor oil packs are easy to make and use, making them accessible for most people to incorporate into their wellness routines. They can be safely used by children, adults, and even the elderly.

Step-by-Step Guide

Materials needed:

- Castor Oil: high-quality cold-pressed castor oil;
- Cotton cloth or flannel: you can buy a pre-made pack with straps that secures around your body, allowing you to carry on with your daily activities or sleep with it on, minimizing any mess, or, you can choose a do-it-yourself castor oil pack using a wool or cotton flannel cloth, preferably organic. Different parts of our body require different pack sizes;
- A plastic wrap / a saran wrap / a plastic bag, or any wrap to prevent staining (even an old towel);
- Heating pad or hot water bottle (optional; pre-made packs are usually designed just to utilize your own body heat);
- Old towel and comfortable clothing. Castor oil stains, so it is preferable to use clothes you do not care for anymore;
- Glass storage container with a lid (for storing the cloth).

Step 1: Prepare the Cloth

Cut a piece of flannel cloth and fold it into 3 or 4 layers to ensure it holds enough oil. Consider the needed size to cover the desired area: for example, if applying the pack to your abdomen, a size about 12x10 inches should suffice.

Step 2: Soak the Cloth

Pour a generous amount of castor oil onto the cloth, ensuring it is thoroughly saturated but not dripping. You can spread the oil evenly by folding the cloth in half and then opening it again. You can always add more if necessary, so proceed gradually to prevent staining your clothes.

If you bought a pre-made pack with straps for easier movement or sleeping, it is suggested to pour 2-3 tablespoons of castor oil in the center of the pack to prevent leakage, then add just 1 tablespoon per use.

Find the optimal adjustment for yourself to minimize mess and enjoy the pack without any inconvenience.

Step 3: Apply the Pack

Apply the castor oil-saturated flannel directly on your skin. Place it on the desired area of your body, such as your liver, abdomen, or joints. The most common placement is on the liver (the right side of the body right below the ribcage) to enhance detoxification. You can place plastic / saran wrap or a thick towel on top of the cotton flannel to avoid getting castor oil on anything else and to prevent the oil from staining your clothes or bedding. If you bought a castor oil pack with straps, you won't need any plastic wrap.

Step 4: Add Heat

Position a heating pad or hot water bottle on top of the plastic-covered cloth. The heat will help the castor oil penetrate deeper into your skin and tissues, and can help relax muscles and soothe pain, enhancing the therapeutic benefits of the pack. If using a heating pad, set it to a comfortable temperature as it must not be too hot.

The goal is mostly to reproduce the warmth of your body: the packs sold for this purpose usually do not require any additional heat source. Anyway, some packs are sold with a microwavable heating pad included that fits in a pocket at the front of the pack wrap. Attention: do not heat castor oil in the microwave!

Step 5: Relax and Allow the Pack to Work

Lie down in a comfortable position and relax. If you want, keep your legs elevated. It's essential to rest while the pack is in place to allow your body to enter a relaxed state and facilitate detoxification and healing.

Leave the pack on for 30-60 minutes, or leave it on overnight for more prolonged benefits.

Step 6: Clean Up

After the session, remove the pack and rub in the excess castor oil if going to sleep, or clean the area with a mild and clean soap and warm water, or with a mix of two tablespoons of baking soda in a quart of water.

If you decide to reuse the material with castor oil on it, it's best to store it in a glass container in the refrigerator or a cool, dark place to prevent it from becoming rancid. You can reuse the cloth several times, adding more oil as needed.

Step 7: Repeat

For best results, repeat the process as needed. Depending on your health goals and how your body responds, you can use castor oil packs several times a week. Most people typically use them two or three times a week, but daily use is also possible.

You can reuse the pack several times (up to 2-3 months), each time adding more oil as needed to keep the pack saturated (usually 1 tbsp of Castor Oil before each use).

Tips for Effective Application

Choose high-quality castor oil

The quality of castor oil is crucial for its therapeutic effectiveness and safety.

High-quality castor oil should be 100% pure, cold-pressed, hexane-free and organic to ensure it is free from harmful chemicals and contaminants. Expeller pressing is also usually safe, as it does not bring the oil over 230°F, thus maintaining its nutrients intact.

Storing castor oil in amber glass bottles is essential as it protects the oil from light exposure, which can degrade its beneficial properties. They also prevents chemical leaching from plastic containers, maintaining the oil's purity and potency.

Store properly

The shelf life of castor oil typically ranges from one to two years, or even more, depending on storage conditions. Key variables that can affect its longevity include exposure to light, heat, and air. To maximize shelf life, store castor oil in a cool, dark place, and ensure the bottle is tightly sealed.

Choose organic wool or cotton flannel

Castor oil packs should only use organic cotton and organic wool, and here's why: castor oil is an excellent carrier oil, meaning it can transport both beneficial substances and harmful chemicals under the skin. Therefore, it is crucial to use clean, organic, unbleached, and dye-free cotton or wool flannel for applications to ensure no harmful substances are introduced.

Many available pre-made packs use organic bamboo, which is not ideal despite being eco-friendly. Bamboo's cellulose fiber is as strong as steel and requires harsh chemicals to break down. These chemicals are not thoroughly washed away to conserve water, because eco-friendly also means that they don't use very much water to clean the material after processing.

Moreover, bamboo is often blended with rayon, which involves the use of phthalates, harmful substances that can disrupt hormones. Therefore, it is crucial to avoid packs made from organic bamboo or rayon blends. Instead, the ideal materials for castor oil packs are organic cotton flannel or organic cotton wool, ensuring the therapy remains effective and free from additional toxins.

Anyway, here a strong recommendation for you: don't let it stop you if you don't have the highest quality cotton piece of flannel, as you will miss all the huge benefits you can get with a castor oil pack!

Choose the material to wrap the pack

If you bought a castor oil pack with straps, no additional wrap is needed. On the other hand, if you opt for a DIY approach you will need some sort of wrap.

Using plastic wrap may seem counterintuitive as it contradicts the plastic-free concept of the flannel or container, so many people prefer using a thick towel on top to avoid staining clothes or bedding, or even parchment paper. Maybe you can ensure that plastic does not come into direct contact with the oil on the skin by placing an extra cotton layer between the soaked flannel and the plastic wrap.

Start slowly

If you are new to castor oil packs, start with shorter sessions (30 minutes) once a week and gradually increase the duration and frequency as your body adjusts.

Consistency is key

Consistent use of castor oil packs can yield better results. It's important to recognize that the advantages of using castor oil packs are often cumulative and require regular use. Consistent application over several weeks or months is generally needed to observe significant improvements, particularly for chronic conditions. Try to include them in your regular wellness routine.

For best results, apply castor oil packs at least four consecutive days per week for a full month. Clients who use them daily report the greatest benefits. Once benefits are experienced, using them once a week to a couple of times a month can maintain these effects. If issues recur, such as digestive distress, painful periods, or inflammation, you can increase frequency. There's flexibility in use; you can adjust based on what feels best for you. If any stomach upset occurs, which is rare, skip a day or two and continue.

Pay attention to your body

Listen to your body and observe how it responds to the castor oil packs. Change how often and how long you use it based on how you feel.

Create a relaxing environment

Enhance the relaxing effect of the castor oil pack by creating a calm environment. Use this time to meditate, listen to soothing music, or practice deep breathing exercises.

Protect your clothing and bedding

Castor oil can stain fabric, so it's best to use old towels and wear comfortable, old clothing that you don't mind getting oily. Alternatively, you can opt for ready-made packs with straps, which are easier and quicker to use.

Follow washing rules

The recommendation is to not wash the pack or the cotton flannel, replacing it every 2 to 3 months based on usage frequency. If you choose to wash it, avoid using a washing machine. Instead, wash it separately by hand using a mild, clean, natural soap with warm water, or a mixture of baking soda and warm water. Additionally, ensure any other towels or clothes used during your castor oil pack session are washed separately.

Store cloth properly

Store the flannel cloth in a glass container in the refrigerator between uses to keep it fresh. Replace the cloth if it starts to smell rancid.

Combine with other wellness practices

Castor oil packs can be part of a broader wellness routine. Consider integrating them with other holistic practices like a healthy diet, regular exercise, and adequate hydration for optimal benefits.

Consult with a Healthcare Provider

If you have any underlying health conditions consult with a healthcare provider before starting the use of castor oil packs to ensure they are safe for you.

Safety Considerations for Castor Oil Use

Castor oil has a long history of use for its therapeutic properties, but like any treatment, it comes with safety considerations that should be observed to ensure its safe and effective use. Here are the main ones:

1. **Allergic reactions**: although rare, some individuals may experience allergic reactions to castor oil, which can include skin rashes, itching, and swelling. Perform a patch test by applying a small amount of castor oil to a patch of skin (such as the inside of your forearm) and wait 24 hours to test for any negative reactions before using it more widely.
2. **Ingestion and digestive issues**: castor oil is a powerful laxative and can cause severe diarrhea, abdominal cramping, and dehydration if ingested in large amounts. Only use castor oil internally under the guidance of a healthcare provider. Follow dosing recommendations strictly. Overuse can lead to nausea, vomiting, and electrolyte imbalances.
3. **Pregnancy**: castor oil can stimulate uterine contractions, which may increase the risk of preterm labor. Therefore, pregnant women should avoid using castor oil both internally and as an external pack.

4. **Heavy menstrual flow**: it is advised that women with heavy menstrual bleeding avoid using castor oil packs during their period. Moreover, if you notice an increase in your menstrual flow and you typically experience heavy bleeding, you should stop using the castor oil pack until your period has ended. For others, these packs can potentially help alleviate menstrual cramps and support the regulation of the menstrual cycle.

5. **Use in children**: children's skin is more sensitive, and they are more susceptible to the effects of medications and treatments. Use castor oil topically in smaller amounts and dilute it if necessary. Avoid using it internally for children without medical advice. Look out for any signs of skin irritation or allergic reaction.

6. **Eye safety**: using non-sterile castor oil near the eyes can introduce infections or cause irritation. Use only sterile, cold-pressed, hexane-free castor oil for eye-related treatments. Ensure hands and applicators are clean.

7. **Skin sensitivity and application**: applying castor oil to broken skin or open wounds can cause irritation and delay healing. Use castor oil on intact skin. For wounds or scars, only apply once the skin has closed, or apply around the area.

8. **Interactions with medications**: castor oil, particularly when ingested, can interact with medications by altering absorption rates. Consult a healthcare provider if you are taking any medications, especially diuretics, heart medications, or other laxatives.

9. **Quality and purity**: impure or adulterated castor oil may contain harmful substances or chemicals. Purchase castor oil from reputable sources. Look for labels indicating cold-pressed, hexane-free, and organic. Avoid products packaged in plastic bottles to prevent chemical leaching. Keep castor oil in a cool, dark location to avoid it becoming rancid.

Different Kinds of Pack

Today, a variety of pre-made castor oil packs are readily available on the market, especially online. Each type addresses different parts of the body and has slightly different characteristics, but they share a common concept: an inner cotton flannel sewn to an outer impermeable layer to prevent oil leakage and staining of clothes, plus adjustable or elastic straps / velcro straps to hold the pack in place. These packs come in different sizes and shapes to better fit the specific body areas they are designed for.

Pack for liver, abdomen, back: usually they have the same shape, which could be described as "oblong" or "rectangular with rounded edges." They are one of the most common and largest kinds of pack.

Pack for pelvis and lower back: this one could be somewhat trapezoidal to cover the entire pelvic area, including the hips.

Pack for eyes: this has the shape of a sleeping mask. It is used to reduce wrinkles around the eyes, promote eye health, enhance the growth of eyelashes and eyebrows, and improve sleep.

Pack for thyroid: usually, the same pack for the eyes can also fit well for the neck.

Packs for breasts: these come as two individual pieces and are somewhat rounded or oval. They are designed with a conic shape to fit the breasts and can be worn under a bra.

Packs for legs, knees, arms: they have different shapes from rounded to rectangular, and different sizes.

Some packs are also designed specifically for wrists and hands.

What if It Does Not Work?

To fully benefit from castor oil packs, it's essential to maintain proper hydration. Castor oil can help move you into a relaxed state, reduce inflammation, and balance your microbiome, but it requires adequate water and minerals to facilitate the removal of toxins from the body.

If you don't notice improvements within the first seven days of using castor oil packs, you should assess your hydration levels. Consider increasing your water intake and possibly incorporating a multi-mineral supplement or electrolytes to enhance absorption and effectiveness.

Electrolytes are charged minerals found in blood, tissues, organs, and bodily fluids. They include magnesium, sodium, potassium, calcium, chloride, and phosphate. These minerals are vital for maintaining water balance, pH levels, and nutrient transport in and out of cells. Electrolytes also ensure proper functioning of muscles, nerves, and organs, and play a crucial role in regulating the nervous system and keeping you hydrated.

Symptoms of electrolyte loss can be fatigue, headaches, low blood pressure, muscle cramps, and nausea. Feeling hungover? You likely need more electrolytes in your system.

If you need to replenish electrolytes in your body to make castor oil packs more effective, you will find 5 easy and tasty recipes that are most popular and appreciated in Chapter 8.

It is also important to understand that, since our bodies function as integrated systems, addressing a single symptom with castor oil without considering underlying health issues may not be effective.

Take, for example, digestive issues. Using castor oil packs might provide immediate relief from constipation by stimulating bowel movements, but the deeper issues like poor dietary habits or an imbalanced gut microbiome also need attention. Incorporating probiotics, making dietary changes, and ensuring proper hydration can support long-term digestive health alongside the use of castor oil packs.

For hormonal imbalances manifesting as irregular menstrual cycles, castor oil packs can alleviate menstrual pain and help hormonal balance. However, it is also vital to address the hormonal dysregulation or thyroid issues that might be causing the symptoms. This comprehensive approach might include dietary adjustments, stress management techniques, and possibly endocrine support, along with the use of castor oil packs.

In the case of skin conditions such as acne, castor oil packs can reduce inflammation and bacterial presence on the skin. But to achieve lasting results, it's necessary to tackle the hormonal imbalances or poor diet that might be at the root of the problem. A holistic skin care routine combined with hormonal treatments and dietary changes, supported by the regular use of castor oil packs, can lead to better skin health.

When dealing with chronic stress and anxiety, castor oil packs can help promote relaxation and reduce cortisol levels, but it's equally important to adopt a lifestyle that includes mindfulness practices, regular exercise, and proper sleep hygiene. These measures, combined with the calming effects of castor oil packs, can significantly improve overall well-being.

By integrating castor oil packs into a broader, holistic health strategy, we address both symptoms and root causes, promoting overall well-being and ensuring a more effective and sustainable approach to health.

Stress Reduction and Improved Sleep

Using a castor oil pack on your abdomen, or even as an eye compress, offers significant stress relief. The calming properties of castor oil, combined with the warmth and gentle pressure of the pack, help lower cortisol levels. This reduction in cortisol subsequently increases melatonin production, fostering relaxation and promoting deep, restorative sleep.

As we learned, the specific softness and gentle pressure from the pack stimulates specific sensory receptors in the skin, that are crucial in sending signals to the brain that are interpreted as soothing and calming. The stimulation of the **vagus nerve** in the parasympathetic nervous system triggers a relaxation response and promotes the release of **oxytocin** and **dopamine**.

Melatonin production is indirectly linked to them. While melatonin production is primarily driven by the light-dark cycle and the pineal gland, oxytocin and dopamine play supporting roles in creating the optimal conditions for melatonin synthesis and overall sleep regulation: **Oxytocin** reduces stress and promotes relaxation, helping to lower cortisol levels, which can interfere with melatonin production, and induces a sense of calm and security, aiding in the transition to sleep; **Dopamine** regulates mood, helping reduce anxiety and depressive symptoms, which are known to disrupt sleep.

Together, these neurotransmitters create an environment conducive to the natural rise of melatonin levels in the evening, facilitating the onset of sleep.

Castor Oil and Overall Wellness

In today's fast-paced society, embracing a holistic approach to health is essential. A holistic perspective integrates mind, body, and spirit, emphasizing balance and wellness through lifestyle, diet, mental health, and natural remedies, thus fostering resilience and enhancing life quality.

Castor oil supports both physical and mental health, as its anti-inflammatory properties and ability to shift the body from stress to relaxation are key. Activation of the parasympathetic nervous system via castor oil packs slows heart rate and breathing, improves immune response, and promotes cell regeneration. It reduces stress hormones, decreases inflammation, promotes nutrient absorption and effective digestion. These processes also aids mental clarity and emotional stability, which are vital for achieving a better quality of life, fostering a sense of fulfillment and truly living life to its fullest.

CHAPTER 8
CASTOR OIL RECIPES

Castor oil is a powerful and versatile ingredient that can work wonders on its own, thanks to its potent properties that benefit the body in numerous ways. Its rich composition makes it a staple in natural beauty and wellness routines, capable of providing deep hydration, promoting hair growth, soothing the skin, and delivering therapeutic properties that enhance our health.

While castor oil alone can deliver impressive results, it is also an excellent carrier oil due to its unique chemical structure and molecular weight. This makes it highly effective at enhancing the properties of other ingredients, whether they are essential oils, vegetable oils, or other natural actives, thereby boosting the overall effectiveness of the treatment.

In this chapter we will cater to those who enjoy the creativity and experimentation of DIY recipes and will explore some of the most popular and effective recipes that are perfect for a variety of uses. We kept them simple and easy because we know most people don't have a lot of time or want to buy a bunch of ingredients. With just a few natural items, you can achieve great results and use them in multiple ways.

For recipes involving castor oil packs, the quantities suggested are for a pre-made pack with straps, allowing you to wear it under your clothes during the day or while sleeping overnight. If you use a cotton flannel, you may need a greater quantity to completely soak the cloth. Just follow your preferences and adjust the quantities as needed. You can refer again to Chapter 7 for details on using packs.

Castor Oil and Orange Juice Cocktail

This recipe has the purpose of making the ingestion of castor oil orally less unpleasant. Since it is the most commonly used, it is probably the most effective!

INGREDIENTS

- 1 to 2 tablespoons (15 to 30 ml) of pure castor oil (be sure to stick to the usage guidelines in Chapter 3)
- 1/2 (half) cup of fresh orange juice (or any preferred juice)
- 1 teaspoon of honey – alternatively maple syrup (optional, if you want to add sweetness)
- A pinch of salt (optional, helps with taste)

INSTRUCTIONS

1. Pour the measured dose of castor oil into a small glass. Add the fresh orange juice to the glass. The strong flavor of orange juice helps to mask the taste of castor oil. If desired, add a teaspoon of honey or maple syrup for extra sweetness and a pinch of salt to further improve the taste.
2. Stir the mixture thoroughly until the castor oil is well blended with the juice. This helps to evenly distribute the oil and make it easier to swallow.
3. Drink the mixture quickly in one go. The faster you drink it, the less you will notice the taste of the castor oil.
4. To completely get rid of the taste, follow up by drinking a small glass of plain juice or water immediately after.

Ginger-Lavender Constipation Relief Castor Oil Pack

Ginger has warming properties and can help to stimulate digestion and improve circulation, making it beneficial for relieving constipation. **Lavender** oil is known for its calming and anti-inflammatory properties, which can help to reduce abdominal discomfort and promote relaxation during the treatment.

INGREDIENTS

- 3 tablespoons castor oil
- 1 teaspoon grated fresh ginger or 1/2 teaspoon (half a teaspoon) ginger powder
- 2-4 drops lavender essential oil

INSTRUCTIONS

1. Warm the castor oil slightly and add the lavender essential oil
2. If using grated fresh ginger, place the grated ginger in a small piece of cheesecloth or a fine strainer. Squeeze out the ginger juice into the oil mixture and discard the pulp. Alternatively, you can let the grated ginger infuse in the oil mixture for a few hours and then strain it out. If using ginger powder, simply add it to the oil mixture and mix well.
3. Apply the mixture to the pack.

Lemon and Lavender Detox Castor Oil Pack

Lemon essential oil detoxifies and cleanses the body, boosts the immune system, and improves circulation. **Lavender** essential oil soothes and calms the mind and body, reduces stress, and promotes relaxation.

INGREDIENTS

- 3 tablespoons castor oil
- 5 drops lemon essential oil
- 5 drops lavender essential oil

INSTRUCTIONS

1. Mix the essential oils with the castor oil
2. Apply the mixture to the pack.

Rosemary and Ginger Detox Castor Oil Pack

Rosemary essential oil stimulates circulation, detoxifies the body, and improves digestion. **Ginger** enhances circulation, reduces inflammation, and aids in digestion.

INGREDIENTS

- 3 tablespoons castor oil
- 5 drops rosemary essential oil
- 1 tablespoon grated fresh ginger or 5 drops ginger essential oil

INSTRUCTIONS

1. Mix the castor oil with the rosemary essential oil and grated ginger or ginger essential oil
2. Apply the mixture to the pack.

Turmeric and Epsom Salt Detox Castor Oil Pack

Turmeric has anti-inflammatory and antioxidant properties, helps detoxify the body, and supports liver health. **Epsom salt** aids in drawing out toxins, reducing inflammation, improving circulation, relaxing muscles, and enhancing overall skin health, contributing to a more effective and soothing detoxification process.

INGREDIENTS

- 3 tablespoons castor oil
- 1 teaspoon turmeric powder or 5 drops turmeric essential oil
- 1 tablespoon Epsom salt

INSTRUCTIONS

1. Dissolve the Epsom salt in a small amount of warm water.
2. Mix the castor oil with the turmeric powder or turmeric essential oil and the dissolved Epsom salt until well combined.
3. Apply the mixture to the pack.

Lavender and Eucalyptus Detox Castor Oil Pack

Lavender essential oil soothes and calms the mind and body, reduces stress, and promotes relaxation. **Eucalyptus** essential oil detoxifies, reduces inflammation, and enhances respiratory function.

INGREDIENTS

- 3 tablespoons castor oil
- 5 drops lavender essential oil
- 5 drops eucalyptus essential oil

INSTRUCTIONS

1. Mix the essential oils with the castor oil
2. Apply the mixture to the pack.

LYMPHATIC DRAINAGE

Castor Oil and Ginger Pack

Ginger stimulates circulation and has anti-inflammatory properties, helping the lymphatic system perform its duties.

INGREDIENTS

- 3 tablespoons castor oil
- 1 tablespoon grated fresh ginger or 5 drops ginger essential oil

INSTRUCTIONS

3. Mix the castor oil with grated ginger or ginger essential oil
4. Apply the mixture to the pack.

Lemon and Grapefruit Essential Oil Massage Blend

Lemon essential oil aids in detoxification and stimulates the lymphatic system, while **grapefruit** essential oil is known for its lymphatic-stimulating properties.

INGREDIENTS

- 3 tablespoons castor oil
- 5 drops lemon essential oil
- 2-3 drops grapefruit essential oil

INSTRUCTIONS

1. Mix the castor oil with the lemon and grapefruit essential oils.
2. Massage the blend gently into the lymphatic areas, using upward strokes towards the heart to promote drainage.
3. Repeat this massage 2-3 times a week for best results.

Rosemary and Castor Oil Lymphatic Massage Oil

Rosemary essential oil improves circulation and supports lymphatic drainage when used in a good body massage.

INGREDIENTS

- 3 tablespoons castor oil
- 5 drops rosemary essential oil

INSTRUCTIONS

1. Mix the castor oil with rosemary essential oil.
2. Use the mixture to massage the lymphatic areas with gentle, circular motions. You can use a body brush with natural bristles for increased effectiveness.
3. Perform the massage 2-3 times a week to support lymphatic drainage.

Eucalyptus and Castor Oil Pack

Eucalyptus essential oil is known for its antiviral and antibacterial properties, and it helps clear respiratory pathways.

INGREDIENTS

- 3 tablespoons castor oil
- 5 drops eucalyptus essential oil

INSTRUCTIONS

1. Mix the castor oil with eucalyptus essential oil.
2. Apply the mixture to the pack.

Tea Tree and Ginger Massage Oil

Tea tree oil has strong antimicrobial properties that can help fight infections. **Ginger** boosts circulation and has anti-inflammatory properties.

INGREDIENTS

- 3 tablespoons castor oil
- 2-3 drops ginger essential oil or 1/2 teaspoon (half a teaspoon) ginger powder
- 2-3 drops tea tree oil

INSTRUCTIONS

1. Mix the castor oil, tea tree oil, and ginger powder or essential oil.
2. Use the mixture to massage the lymphatic areas with gentle, circular motions.
3. Perform the massage 2-3 times a week.

Lavender and Cayenne Castor Oil Pack

Lavender essential oil helps to reduce pain and inflammation and promotes relaxation. **Cayenne pepper** (Capsaicin) is known to reduce pain by depleting substance P[42], a compound that transmits pain signals.

INGREDIENTS

- 3 tablespoons castor oil
- 5 drops lavender essential oil
- 1/2 teaspoon (half a teaspoon) cayenne pepper powder

INSTRUCTIONS

1. Mix the castor oil with lavender essential oil and cayenne pepper powder.
2. Apply the mixture to the pack.

---

42   Altınterim, B. (2013). Cayenne, Capsaicin and Substance-P. *ResearchGate*.

Turmeric and Lemon Castor Oil Pack

Turmeric has curcumin, a compound with strong anti-inflammatory and antioxidant effects. **Lemon** essential oil is rich in vitamin C, it boosts immunity and detoxifies the body.

INGREDIENTS

- 3 tablespoons castor oil
- 1/2 teaspoon (half a teaspoon) to 3/4 teaspoon (three-quarters of a teaspoon) turmeric powder
- 4 drops lemon essential oil

INSTRUCTIONS

1. Mix the castor oil with turmeric powder and lemon essential oil.
2. Apply the mixture to the pack.

Rosemary and Peppermint Massage Oil

Rosemary essential oil enhances circulation and has antimicrobial properties. **Peppermint** essential oil helps clear the respiratory system and has antibacterial properties.

INGREDIENTS

- 3 tablespoons castor oil
- 5 drops rosemary essential oil
- 2-3 drops peppermint essential oil

INSTRUCTIONS

1. Mix the castor oil, rosemary essential oil, and peppermint essential oil.
2. Use the mixture to massage the chest and back areas to support respiratory health.
3. Perform the massage 2-3 times a week.

PAIN RELIEF AND INFLAMMATION REMEDIES

Eucalyptus and Wintergreen Pack

Eucalyptus essential oil contains anti-inflammatory and analgesic properties that help to relieve pain and reduce inflammation. It also provides a cooling sensation that can ease muscle soreness. **Wintergreen** essential oil contains methyl salicylate, which has strong analgesic and anti-inflammatory properties. It is frequently utilized to alleviate muscle and joint discomfort.

INGREDIENTS

- 3 tablespoons castor oil
- 5-10 drops eucalyptus essential oil
- 5 drops wintergreen essential oil

INSTRUCTIONS

1. Mix the castor oil with the eucalyptus and wintergreen essential oils
2. Apply the mixture to the pack.

Peppermint and Ginger Massage Oil

Peppermint essential oil contains menthol, which offers a cooling sensation and helps to soothe pain and reduce inflammation. **Ginger** has warming properties and anti-inflammatory effects.

INGREDIENTS

- 3 tablespoons castor oil
- 5 drops peppermint essential oil
- 1 tablespoon grated fresh ginger or 5 drops ginger essential oil

INSTRUCTIONS

1. Mix the castor oil with the peppermint essential oil.
2. Add the grated fresh ginger or the ginger essential oil and mix well.
3. Apply a small amount of the oil to your hands and gently massage it into the desired area, using circular motions.
4. Perform the massage 2-3 times a week.

Turmeric and Arnica Castor Oil Balm

Turmeric has curcumin, a compound with strong anti-inflammatory and antioxidant effects. **Arnica** is known for its ability to reduce pain, swelling, and bruising.

INGREDIENTS

- 3 tablespoons castor oil
- 1/2 teaspoon (half a teaspoon) to 3/4 teaspoon (three-quarters of a teaspoon) turmeric powder
- 1 1/2 teaspoons (one and a half teaspoons) arnica oil or gel

INSTRUCTIONS

1. Mix the castor oil with turmeric powder and arnica oil or gel.
2. Massage the balm gently onto the affected areas.
3. For optimal results, use this treatment 2-3 times per week.

Healing and Antiseptic Ointment

This simple yet powerful recipe combines the healing properties of castor oil, honey, and essential oils to create an effective ointment for minor cuts, scrapes, and wounds.

Beeswax creates a protective barrier, preventing infection and keeping the area moist. **Honey** offers antibacterial properties and aids in tissue regeneration and **tea tree** essential oil prevents infection with its strong antiseptic properties. **Lavender** essential oil promotes healing and reduces pain and inflammation.

INGREDIENTS

- 3 tablespoons castor oil
- 1 1/2 tablespoons (one and a half tablespoons) beeswax
- 1 1/2 teaspoons (one and a half teaspoons) honey
- 4 drops tea tree essential oil
- 4 drops lavender essential oil

INSTRUCTIONS

1. Melt the beeswax in a double boiler or a heatproof bowl over a pot of simmering water, gently melt the beeswax until it becomes liquid.
2. Add the castor oil and honey to the melted beeswax and stir well to combine. Remove the mixture from heat and let it cool slightly.
3. Once the mixture has cooled but is still liquid, add the tea tree essential oil and lavender essential oil. Stir thoroughly to ensure all ingredients are well incorporated.
4. Pour the mixture into clean, sterilized glass container. Allow the ointment to cool and solidify completely before capping the container.
5. Clean the area with mild soap and water, then apply a thin layer of the ointment to the cut, scrape, or wound. Cover with a bandage if needed.
6. Use 2-3 times a day or as needed until the wound is healed. It can be stored and used for about 6 months to 1 year if stored properly.

ANTI-INFLAMMATORY AND ANTIBACTERIAL

Healing Power Salve

This is an anti-inflammatory and antibacterial ointment which is ideal for treating fungal nail infections, ringworm, bug bites, warts, and various skin irritations. **Tea tree** oil is antibacterial, antifungal, antiviral, and anti-inflammatory. **Baking soda** has got antifungal, antibacterial, and exfoliating properties.

INGREDIENTS

- 3 tablespoons castor oil
- 3-5 drops tea tree oil
- baking soda in a sufficient quantity

INSTRUCTIONS

1. Mix castor oil, tea tree oil and a little bit of baking soda in a small container (choose only glass containers).
2. Mix all the ingredients together until the consistency becomes a paste. If it is too liquid, add more baking soda gradually.
3. Use it as often as you like on the affected areas.
4. It can be stored and used for months if stored properly.

WOMEN'S HEALTH

Comfort Relaxation Pack

Lavender essential oil is known for its calming and soothing properties, lavender oil helps to reduce stress and promote relaxation. **Chamomile** essential oil is renowned for its relaxing and anti-inflammatory properties. It helps to soothe muscle cramps and promote a sense of well-being.

INGREDIENTS

- 3 tablespoons castor oil
- 5 drops lavender essential oil
- 5 drops chamomile essential oil

INSTRUCTIONS

1. Mix the castor oil with the lavender and chamomile essential oils.
2. Apply the mixture to the pack.
3. If you want, use a hot water bottle or heating pad to keep the pack warm.

Refreshing Massage Elixir

Clary sage essential oil has antispasmodic properties that can help relieve menstrual cramps and balance hormones. **Peppermint** essential oil provides a cooling sensation and relieves pain and muscle spasms.

INGREDIENTS

- 3 tablespoons castor oil
- 4 drops clary sage essential oil
- 2 drops peppermint essential oil

INSTRUCTIONS

1. Mix the castor oil, clary sage essential oil, and peppermint essential oil.
2. Use the mixture to massage the lower abdomen and lower back in gentle, circular motions.
3. Perform the massage as needed for relief.

Warmth Healing Pack

Ginger not only stimulates circulation and has anti-inflammatory properties, but also possesses warming properties that can help soothe cramps. **Cayenne pepper** enhances the warming effect and helps reducing pain.

INGREDIENTS

- 3 tablespoons castor oil
- 1/2 teaspoon (half a teaspoon) to 3/4 teaspoon (three-quarters of a teaspoon) ginger powder or 5 drops ginger essential oil
- 1/4 teaspoon (one-quarter of a teaspoon) cayenne pepper powder

INSTRUCTIONS

1. Mix the castor oil with the ginger powder or ginger essential oil and cayenne pepper powder
2. Apply the mixture to the pack.
3. If you want, use a hot water bottle or heating pad to keep the pack warm.

Serenity Balance Castor Oil Pack

Rose essential oil has calming and uplifting properties. It helps to balance hormones, reduce stress, and promote emotional well-being. **Geranium** essential oil is known for its balancing and calming effects. It helps to alleviate stress, balance hormones, and improve mood.

INGREDIENTS

- 3 tablespoons castor oil
- 5 drops rose essential oil
- 5 drops geranium essential oil

INSTRUCTIONS

1. Mix the castor oil with the rose and geranium essential oils.
2. Apply the mixture to the pack.
3. If you want, use a hot water bottle or heating pad to keep the pack warm.

Bergamot and Ylang Ylang Castor Oil Pack

Bergamot essential oil is known for its calming and uplifting properties and helps to alleviate anxiety, reduce stress, and improve mood. **Ylang ylang** essential oil is known for its relaxing and sedative properties. It helps to reduce stress, lower blood pressure, and promote a sense of well-being.

INGREDIENTS

- 3 tablespoons castor oil
- 5 drops bergamot essential oil
- 5 drops ylang ylang essential oil

INSTRUCTIONS

1. Mix the castor oil with the bergamot and ylang ylang essential oils.
2. Apply the mixture to the cloth or pack.

Aromatherapy Massage

Chamomile essential oil is known for its calming effects, while **sandalwood** essential oil helps promote mental clarity and relaxation. When combined with castor oil, these essential oils create a powerful blend that eases muscle tension and enhances overall relaxation, making this massage ideal for stress relief and mental wellness.

INGREDIENTS

- 3 tablespoons castor oil
- 4 drops chamomile essential oil
- 2 drops sandalwood essential oil

INSTRUCTIONS

1. Mix the castor oil with chamomile and sandalwood essential oils.
2. Use the blend to give yourself or someone else a gentle, calming massage, focusing on the shoulders, neck, and feet.
3. Perform this massage in a quiet, comfortable environment to enhance relaxation.

Stress-Relief Bath

Epsom salt is famous for its muscle-relaxing and detoxifying properties, while **rosemary** and **lavender** essential oils add a soothing and calming effect. Mixing these with castor oil creates a bath that not only relaxes muscles but also calms the mind, making it perfect for relieving stress and promoting a sense of well-being.

INGREDIENTS

- 1/4 (one-quarter) cup castor oil
- 1 cup Epsom salt
- 10 drops rosemary essential oil
- 10 drops lavender essential oil

INSTRUCTIONS

1. Run a warm bath and add the Epsom salt, rosemary essential oil, and lavender essential oil.
2. Mix the castor oil into the bathwater.
3. Soak in the bath for 20-30 minutes, allowing the ingredients to soothe your muscles and mind.

Mindfulness Ritual

Frankincense essential oil is known for its ability to promote mental clarity and relaxation. Combined with the anti-inflammatory properties of castor oil, this blend is perfect for enhancing meditation and mindfulness practices, helping to reduce stress and improve mental focus.

INGREDIENTS

- 3 tablespoons castor oil
- 5 drops frankincense essential oil

INSTRUCTIONS

1. Mix the castor oil with the frankincense essential oil.
2. Apply a small amount of the mixture to your temples and the back of your neck.
3. Practice deep breathing or meditation for 10-15 minutes, allowing the scent and therapeutic properties to calm your mind and body.

Sleep Aid Blend

Cedarwood essential oil is excellent for promoting restful sleep, while **lavender** essential oil helps reduce anxiety and stress. When combined with castor oil, these essential oils create a powerful blend that supports relaxation and restful sleep, making it an effective remedy for stress and insomnia.

INGREDIENTS

- 3 tablespoons castor oil
- 5 drops cedarwood essential oil
- 5 drops lavender essential oil

INSTRUCTIONS

1. Mix the castor oil with cedarwood and lavender essential oils.
2. Apply a small amount to the soles of your feet and massage gently before bedtime.
3. This blend can help promote restful sleep and reduce stress.

CASTOR OIL FOR CHILDREN

Relaxing Massage for Children

Creating a peaceful bedtime routine is essential for children's overall well-being, and a soothing massage can work wonders in helping them unwind and relax. This recipe combines the deeply hydrating and calming properties of castor oil with the gentle, nourishing benefits of **sweet almond oil**. Adding a few drops of **chamomile** essential oil can further enhance the relaxing effects, making it an optional but valuable addition.

INGREDIENTS

- 2 tablespoons castor oil
- 1 tablespoon sweet almond oil
- Chamomile essential oil (optional)

INSTRUCTIONS

1. Mix the oils in a small dark glass bottle.
2. Warm a small amount of the oil mixture between your hands.
3. Gently massage the oil onto the child's skin, focusing on areas that need relaxation like legs and feet, tummy (abdomen), and forehead and temples, to help them unwind before bedtime.

Diaper Rash Soothing Balm with Castor Oil

Coconut oil deeply moisturizes and protects the skin with its antibacterial and antifungal properties. Shea butter nourishes and heals the skin with its rich vitamins and moisturizing properties. Chamomile essential oil calms irritated skin and reduces redness with its anti-inflammatory properties.

INGREDIENTS

- 2 tablespoons castor oil
- 2 tablespoons coconut oil
- 1 tablespoon shea butter
- 5 drops chamomile essential oil (optional)

INSTRUCTIONS

1. In a double boiler, melt the coconut oil and shea butter over low heat until fully liquefied.
2. Remove from heat and let the mixture cool slightly.
3. Pour in the castor oil and mix until thoroughly blended.
4. If using, add the chamomile essential oil and mix thoroughly.
5. Pour the mixture into a clean glass container and let it solidify at room temperature or in the refrigerator.
6. Once solidified, take a small amount and gently apply it to the affected area on the baby's skin.
7. Use as needed to soothe and protect against diaper rash.

Calming Bedtime Balm for Children

Coconut oil deeply moisturizes and protects the skin with its antibacterial and antifungal properties. **Shea butter** nourishes and heals the skin with its rich vitamins and moisturizing properties. **Lavender** essential oil is known for its calming and relaxing properties and helps to promote better sleep and reduce anxiety. **Chamomile** essential oil has soothing and calming properties that help to relax the child and promote restful sleep.

INGREDIENTS

- 2 tablespoons castor oil
- 2 tablespoons coconut oil
- 1 tablespoon shea butter
- 5 drops lavender essential oil
- 5 drops chamomile essential oil

INSTRUCTIONS

1. In a double boiler, melt the coconut oil and shea butter over low heat until fully liquefied.
2. Remove from heat and let the mixture cool slightly.
3. Pour in the castor oil and mix until thoroughly blended.
4. Add the lavender and chamomile essential oils and mix thoroughly.
5. Transfer the mixture to a clean container and allow it to solidify either at room temperature or in the refrigerator.
6. Once solidified, take a small amount and gently apply it to the child's chest, back, or feet before bedtime to help promote relaxation and better sleep.

Coconut Oil Growth Serum

Known for its moisturizing and nourishing properties, **coconut** oil helps to condition the hair, making it softer and shinier. It also contains fatty acids that penetrate the hair shaft, providing deep hydration. **Vitamin E** is an antioxidant that helps to repair and build tissue and can improve hair health by preventing breakage and promoting stronger, healthier growth.

INGREDIENTS

- 1/2 teaspoon (half a teaspoon) castor oil
- 1/2 teaspoon (half a teaspoon) coconut oil
- 5 drops of vitamin E oil

INSTRUCTIONS

1. In a small, clean glass container, mix the castor oil and coconut oil until well combined.
2. If using, add the vitamin E oil and stir until fully incorporated.
3. Using a clean mascara wand or cotton swab, apply the mixture to your eyelashes and eyebrows, making sure to coat them thoroughly but not excessively.
4. Leave it on overnight and wash off with warm water in the morning.
5. Use this serum daily for best results.

Aloe Vera Gel Growth Serum

Aloe vera gel is known for its soothing and moisturizing properties and helps to condition the hair and promote a healthy scalp. It also contains enzymes that repair dead skin cells, creating a healthy environment for hair growth. **Rosemary** essential oil stimulates blood circulation to the hair follicles, promoting hair growth. It also has antibacterial properties that help to keep the scalp clean and healthy.

INGREDIENTS

- 1/2 teaspoon (half a teaspoon) castor oil
- 1/2 teaspoon (half a teaspoon) aloe vera gel
- 2-3 drops rosemary essential oil

INSTRUCTIONS

1. In a small, clean container, mix the castor oil and aloe vera gel until well combined.
2. Add the rosemary essential oil and stir until fully incorporated.
3. Using a clean mascara wand or cotton swab, apply the mixture to your eyelashes and eyebrows, ensuring even coverage.
4. Leave it on overnight and wash off with warm water in the morning.
5. Use this serum daily for best results.

Aloe Vera and Cucumber Hydrating Mask

Aloe vera is known for its soothing and hydrating properties. It helps to calm irritated skin, reduce inflammation, and provide a moisture boost. **Cucumber** is highly hydrating and contains antioxidants. It helps to cool and refresh the skin, reducing puffiness and soothing irritation. **Rose water** is a natural toner that balances the skin's pH, hydrates, and reduces redness and inflammation. It also provides a gentle, pleasant fragrance.

INGREDIENTS

- 1 tablespoon castor oil
- 2 tablespoons aloe vera gel
- 1 tablespoon cucumber juice
- 1 teaspoon rose water

INSTRUCTIONS

1. Place the grated ginger in a small piece of cheesecloth or a fine strainer. Squeeze out the ginger juice and discard the pulp.
2. Mix the castor oil, aloe vera gel, cucumber juice and rose water in a small bowl until well combined.
3. Apply the mixture to your face
4. Leave it on for 15-20 minutes.
5. Rinse off with warm water and gently dry your skin with a towel.
6. Follow with your favorite moisturizer.

Honey and Oatmeal Hydrating Facial

This facial combines moisturizing, exfoliating, and healing properties, making it effective for hydrating and rejuvenating the skin while providing gentle exfoliation. **Honey** acts as a natural humectant, because it attracts and retains moisture. It also has antibacterial and antioxidant properties, helping to heal and protect the skin. **Oatmeal** is soothing and anti-inflammatory. It helps to gently exfoliate the skin, removing dead skin cells and promoting a smoother complexion. **Yogurt** has lactic acid that softly exfoliates and brightens the skin. It also offers extra hydration and a cooling sensation.

INGREDIENTS

- 1 tablespoon castor oil
- 1 tablespoon raw honey
- 1 tablespoon finely ground oatmeal
- 1 teaspoon yogurt (optional for extra hydration)

INSTRUCTIONS

1. Combine the castor oil, honey, oatmeal, and yogurt (if using) in a small bowl and mix well.
2. Apply the mixture evenly to your face.
3. Let it sit for 15-20 minutes.
4. Rinse off with warm water and gently dry your skin with a towel.
5. Apply your regular moisturizer.

Avocado and Banana Hydrating Mask

This mask is highly nourishing and hydrating, perfect for revitalizing dry and dull skin. **Avocado** is rich in vitamins E and C, healthy fats, and antioxidants. It deeply moisturizes, nourishes, and repairs the skin. **Banana** is packed with vitamins A, B, and E, as well as potassium. It helps to hydrate and soften the skin, reducing the appearance of dryness and fine lines. **Lemon** juice is rich in vitamin C and has brightening properties. It helps to even out skin tone and reduce dark spots, though it should be used sparingly to avoid irritation. **Honey** adds moisture, heals, and protects the skin with its antibacterial and antioxidant properties.

INGREDIENTS

- 1 tablespoon castor oil
- 1/2 (half) ripe avocado
- 1/2 (half) ripe banana
- 1 teaspoon lemon juice (for added brightness)
- 1 teaspoon honey

INSTRUCTIONS

1. Mash the avocado and banana in a bowl until they become a smooth paste.
2. Add the castor oil, lemon juice, and honey to the mashed mixture and mix well.
3. Apply the mixture to your face, covering all areas evenly.
4. Leave the mask on for 20-25 minutes.
5. Rinse off with warm water and gently dry your skin with a towel.
6. Apply a moisturizer for more hydration.

Tea Tree Oil and Aloe Vera Acne Treatment

Tea tree oil is known for its potent antibacterial and anti-inflammatory properties and helps to kill acne-causing bacteria and reduce redness and swelling. **Aloe vera** gel soothes and hydrates the skin while providing anti-inflammatory benefits. It aids in soothing irritated skin and encourages healing.

INGREDIENTS

- 1 tablespoon castor oil
- 2-3 drops tea tree oil
- 1 tablespoon aloe vera gel

INSTRUCTIONS

1. Mix the castor oil, tea tree oil, and aloe vera gel in a small bowl until well combined.
2. Spread the mixture on your face, concentrating on areas prone to acne.
3. Leave it on for 15-20 minutes.
4. Rinse off with warm water and gently dry your skin with a towel.
5. For optimal results, use this treatment 2-3 times per week.

Castor Oil and Green Clay Spot Treatment

Green clay is known for its detoxifying and oil-absorbing properties and helps to draw out impurities and excess oil from the skin, reducing the likelihood of clogged pores and breakouts. **Apple cider vinegar** has acetic acid, which possesses antibacterial and antifungal qualities. It helps to balance the skin's PH and reduce the appearance of acne. **Aloe vera** gel soothes and hydrates the skin while providing anti-inflammatory benefits. It soothes irritated skin and supports the healing process.

INGREDIENTS

- 1 tablespoon castor oil
- 1 tablespoon green clay
- 1 teaspoon apple cider vinegar (optional if you want more antibacterial qualities)
- 1 teaspoon aloe vera gel (optional for soothing effects)

INSTRUCTIONS

1. In a small, clean container, mix the green clay and castor oil until they form a smooth paste.
2. If using, add the apple cider vinegar and aloe vera gel to the mixture and stir until well combined.
3. Using a clean cotton swab or your fingertip, apply a small amount of the mixture directly to the acne spots.
4. Leave it on for 15-20 minutes or until it fully dries.
5. Rinse off with warm water and gently dry your skin with a towel.
6. Use this spot treatment as needed, up to twice daily for best results.

Eczema and Psoriasis Soothing Blend

Calendula oil is known for its healing properties, it helps to reduce inflammation and promote skin regeneration. **Chamomile** essential oil is calming and anti-inflammatory, it soothes irritated skin and helps reduce the symptoms of eczema and psoriasis.

INGREDIENTS

- 1 tablespoon castor oil
- 1 tablespoon calendula oil
- 5 drops chamomile essential oil

INSTRUCTIONS

1. In a small bottle, mix castor oil, calendula oil, and chamomile essential oil.
2. Apply a small amount to the affected areas and gently massage it in.
3. Use this blend 2-3 times daily to soothe and heal the skin.

Anti-Aging Serum

Jojoba oil closely mimics the skin's natural sebum, making it an excellent moisturizer. It is non-comedogenic and helps to balance oil production, keeping the skin hydrated and reducing the signs of aging. **Rosehip** oil is high in essential fatty acids and vitamins A and C and promotes skin regeneration and improves skin texture. It helps to reduce the appearance of scars, fine lines, and hyperpigmentation, giving the skin a more even tone and youthful glow. **Frankincense** essential oil is known for its powerful anti-aging properties and helps to improve skin elasticity, reduce the appearance of wrinkles, and promote cell regeneration. It also has anti-inflammatory properties that soothe and protect the skin. **Vitamin E** oil is an antioxidant that helps to protect the skin from free radical damage. It promotes skin healing and reduces the appearance of fine lines and wrinkles.

INGREDIENTS

- 1 tablespoon castor oil
- 1 tablespoon jojoba oil
- 1 teaspoon rosehip oil
- 5 drops frankincense essential oil
- 2 drops vitamin E oil (optional for added nourishment)

INSTRUCTIONS

1. In a small, clean container, combine the castor oil, jojoba oil, and rosehip oil.
2. Add the frankincense essential oil and vitamin E oil (if using) and mix well.
3. Apply a few drops of the serum to your face and neck, gently massaging it into the skin in upward circular motions.
4. Use this serum nightly before bed for best results.

Nourishing Nail and Cuticle Oil

Jojoba oil mimics the skin's natural oils and provides deep hydration, promoting healthy nails and cuticles. **Vitamin E** oil is an antioxidant that helps to repair and protect the skin and nails, promoting healthy growth and preventing breakage. **Lavender** essential oil has soothing and healing properties that help to nourish and protect the nails and cuticles. **Tea tree** essential oil is known for its antibacterial and antifungal properties and helps to keep the nails and cuticles healthy and free from infections.

INGREDIENTS

- 1 tablespoon castor oil
- 1 tablespoon jojoba oil
- 1 teaspoon vitamin E oil
- 5 drops lavender essential oil
- 5 drops tea tree essential oil

INSTRUCTIONS

1. In a small, clean bottle, combine the castor oil, jojoba oil, and vitamin E oil.
2. Add the lavender and tea tree essential oils.
3. Shake well to mix all ingredients thoroughly.
4. Using a small brush or dropper, apply a small amount of the oil to your nails and cuticles.
5. Massage gently for a few minutes until the oil is absorbed.
6. Use this oil daily for best results.

Shea Butter Hand Cream

This rich hand cream combines the deeply moisturizing properties of castor oil and **shea butter** which is rich in vitamins and fatty acids, and deeply moisturizes and nourishes the skin. **Coconut** oil adds additional moisture and helps protect the skin barrier, while **lavender** essential oil soothes and calms the skin, providing a pleasant aroma.

INGREDIENTS

- 2 tablespoons castor oil
- 2 tablespoons shea butter
- 1 tablespoon coconut oil
- 5 drops lavender essential oil

INSTRUCTIONS

1. In a double boiler, gently melt the shea butter and coconut oil until fully liquefied.
2. Remove from heat and add the castor oil to the melted mixture. Stir well to combine.
3. Stir in the lavender essential oil and blend well.
4. Pour the mixture into a small glass container and let it cool until it solidifies. You can place it in the refrigerator to speed up the process.
5. Apply a small amount of the cream to your hands, massaging it in until fully absorbed. Use daily or as needed to keep your hands soft and hydrated.

Castor Oil and Peppermint Foot Soak

This invigorating foot soak combines the healing properties of castor oil with the refreshing and cooling effects of **peppermint** essential oil. **Epsom salts** help to soothe tired feet and reduce inflammation, making this soak perfect for a relaxing and rejuvenating treatment.

INGREDIENTS

- 1/4 (one-quarter) cup castor oil
- 1/2 (half) cup Epsom salts
- 10 drops peppermint essential oil
- Warm water

INSTRUCTIONS

1. Pour warm water into a basin or foot bath. Add the Epsom salts and stir until dissolved.
2. In a small bowl, combine the castor oil and peppermint essential oil. Pour the oil mixture into the warm water and stir to distribute.
3. Immerse your feet in the solution for 20-30 minutes, letting the ingredients take effect. You can gently massage your feet while soaking to enhance the benefits.
4. After soaking, gently dry your feet with a towel. Apply a moisturizer or additional castor oil to lock in hydration.

Castor Oil and Shea Butter Treatment

Rich in vitamins A, E, and F, **shea butter** deeply moisturizes and nourishes the skin. Its anti-inflammatory and healing properties help to reduce the appearance of scars and stretch marks. **Coconut** oil contains fatty acids that moisturize and nourish the skin. It helps to improve skin barrier function and reduces the appearance of scars and stretch marks. **Lavender** essential oil is known for its calming and healing properties and helps to reduce inflammation and promote skin regeneration.

INGREDIENTS

- 2 tablespoons castor oil
- 2 tablespoons shea butter
- 1 tablespoon coconut oil
- 5 drops lavender essential oil

INSTRUCTIONS

1. Melt the shea butter and coconut oil in a double boiler over low heat until they are fully liquid.
2. Remove from heat and let it cool slightly, then add the castor oil and lavender essential oil. Mix well.
3. Transfer the mixture to a clean container and allow it to solidify either at room temperature or in the refrigerator.
4. Once solidified, take a small amount and massage it into the scar or stretch mark areas in circular motions until fully absorbed.
5. Use this treatment daily for best results.

Castor Oil and Vitamin E Treatment

High in essential fatty acids and vitamins A and C, **rosehip** oil promotes skin regeneration, reduces the appearance of scars, and improves skin texture and tone. **Vitamin E** oil is a powerful antioxidant that helps to protect the skin from free radical damage and promotes healing. It helps to reduce the appearance of scars and stretch marks by improving skin elasticity and hydration. **Frankincense** essential oil is known for its skin-regenerating and anti-inflammatory properties and helps to improve skin tone, reduce the appearance of scars, and promote overall skin health.

INGREDIENTS

- 2 tablespoons castor oil
- 1 tablespoon rosehip oil
- 1 teaspoon vitamin E oil
- 5 drops frankincense essential oil

INSTRUCTIONS

1. In a small, clean container, combine the castor oil, rosehip oil, vitamin E oil, and frankincense essential oil. Mix well.
2. Apply a small amount of the mixture to the scar or stretch mark areas.
3. Massage the oil gently into your skin using circular motions until it is completely absorbed.
4. Use this treatment daily for best results.

Anti-Dandruff Castor Oil Scalp Treatment

Jojoba oil mimics the scalp's natural sebum and helps to balance oil production, moisturize the scalp, and prevent dryness and flakiness. **Tea tree** essential oil, with its potent antibacterial and antifungal properties, is effective in treating dandruff caused by fungal infections. It helps to cleanse the scalp and reduce inflammation. **Peppermint** essential oil is known for its cooling and soothing properties and helps to alleviate itching and irritation associated with dandruff. It also promotes better blood circulation to the scalp, which can enhance overall scalp health.

INGREDIENTS

- 2 tablespoons castor oil
- 1 tablespoon jojoba oil
- 10 drops tea tree essential oil
- 5 drops peppermint essential oil

INSTRUCTIONS

1. In a small container, mix the castor oil, jojoba oil, tea tree essential oil, and peppermint essential oil until well combined.
2. Apply the mixture to your scalp, massaging it in circular motions to ensure even distribution.
3. It can be applied for at least 30 minutes or left on overnight.
4. Rinse thoroughly and shampoo as usual.
5. Use this treatment once or twice a week for best results.

Invigorating Castor Oil Scalp Treatment

Argan oil is rich in essential fatty acids, vitamin E, and antioxidants. It deeply conditions the scalp and hair, adds shine, and promotes healthy hair growth. **Rosemary** essential oil is known for its ability to stimulate hair follicles, increase blood circulation to the scalp, and promote hair growth. It also possesses anti-inflammatory and antimicrobial qualities that maintain scalp health. **Peppermint** essential oil provides a cooling and tingling sensation that invigorates the scalp. It aids in enhancing blood circulation, alleviating inflammation, and calming irritation. Its antimicrobial properties also help maintain scalp health.

INGREDIENTS

- 2 tablespoons castor oil
- 1 tablespoon argan oil
- 10 drops rosemary essential oil
- 5 drops peppermint essential oil

INSTRUCTIONS

1. In a small container, mix the castor oil, argan oil, rosemary essential oil, and peppermint essential oil until well combined.
2. Apply the mixture to your scalp, massaging it in circular motions to stimulate blood flow and ensure even distribution.
3. It can be applied for at least 30 minutes or left on overnight.
4. Rinse thoroughly and shampoo as usual.
5. Use this treatment once or twice a week for best results.

Nourishing Castor Oil Hair Mask

Coconut oil contains fatty acids that penetrate the hair shaft, providing deep conditioning and moisture. It also helps to reduce protein loss and adds shine to the hair. **Honey** isa natural humectant and attracts and retains moisture, keeping the hair hydrated. Its antibacterial properties also promote a healthy scalp. **Avocado** is packed with vitamins A, D, E, and B6, as well as healthy fats, and nourishes and hydrates the hair, promoting softness and shine. **Egg yolk** is rich in proteins, vitamins, and fatty acids. It strengthens the hair, adds moisture, and promotes hair growth. It also helps to repair and nourish damaged hair.

INGREDIENTS

- 2 tablespoons castor oil
- 1 tablespoon coconut oil
- 1 tablespoon honey
- 1 ripe avocado
- 1 egg yolk

INSTRUCTIONS

1. In a small bowl, mash the ripe avocado until it becomes smooth.
2. Add the castor oil, coconut oil, honey, and egg yolk to the avocado and mix until well combined.
3. Apply the mixture to your hair. Concentrate on the roots and ends.
4. Cover your hair with a shower cap for 30-60 minutes.
5. Rinse well with lukewarm water and then shampoo as you normally would.
6. Use this hair mask once a week for best results.

Hydrating Castor Oil Hair Tonic Spray

Argan oil is rich in essential fatty acids, vitamin E, and antioxidants, and deeply conditions and nourishes the hair, making it soft and manageable. **Distilled water** acts as the base for the tonic, providing hydration and ensuring the other ingredients are evenly distributed. **Aloe vera** juice has moisturizing and soothing qualities. It helps to hydrate the hair and scalp, promoting healthy hair growth and reducing frizz. **Lavender** essential oil adds a pleasant fragrance and has soothing properties that help to calm the scalp. It also promotes hair growth and helps to maintain a healthy scalp. **Rose** essential oil provides a delightful floral scent and helps to moisturize and nourish the hair. Its soothing properties are beneficial for the scalp.

INGREDIENTS

- 1 tablespoon castor oil
- 1 tablespoon argan oil
- 1 cup distilled water
- 2 tablespoons aloe vera juice
- 10 drops lavender essential oil
- 5 drops rose essential oil

INSTRUCTIONS

1. In a spray bottle, combine the distilled water and aloe vera juice.
2. Add the castor oil and argan oil to the mixture.
3. Add the lavender and rose essential oils. Shake the bottle well.
4. Spray the tonic onto your hair, focusing on the ends and any dry areas.
5. Use daily or as needed for hydration and shine.

ELECTROLITES INTEGRATION

Here are five popular and easy recipes for electrolyte supplementation, which you can make at home to stay hydrated and replenish essential minerals. To fully benefit from castor oil packs, remember it's essential to maintain proper hydration.

Basic Electrolyte Drink

This basic recipe provides sodium for fluid balance, potassium from the lemon, and carbohydrates from honey for quick energy. To fully benefit from castor oil packs, it's essential to maintain proper hydration and adequate mineral levels to facilitate the removal of toxins from the body..

INGREDIENTS

- 1 liter (4 cups) of water
- Juice of 1 lemon
- 1/4 teaspoon (one-quarter of a teaspoon) of salt (preferably Himalayan pink salt or sea salt)
- 2 tablespoons of honey or 100% pure maple syrup

INSTRUCTIONS

1. Squeeze the juice of one lemon into the water.
2. Add the salt and honey (or maple syrup), and stir until fully dissolved.
3. Chill in the refrigerator before consuming.

Coconut Water Electrolyte Drink

Coconut water is naturally high in potassium, while the orange juice adds additional potassium and vitamin C. The salt replenishes sodium lost through sweat.

INGREDIENTS

- 2 cups of coconut water
- 1/2 (half) cup of fresh orange juice
- 1/4 teaspoon (one-quarter of a teaspoon) of salt

INSTRUCTIONS

1. Mix all ingredients in a pitcher.
2. Stir well and chill before drinking.

Adrenal Cocktail

This drink is packed with potassium from the coconut water, orange juice, and cream of tartar, helping to support adrenal function and maintain electrolyte balance.

INGREDIENTS

- 1 cup of coconut water
- 1/2 (half) cup of orange juice
- 1/4 teaspoon (one-quarter of a teaspoon) of cream of tartar
- A pinch of salt

INSTRUCTIONS

1. Mix all ingredients thoroughly.
2. Serve chilled.

Maple Syrup Electrolyte Drink

This recipe uses maple syrup, which is a natural source of minerals, and lime juice, which provides vitamin C and potassium. The salt helps to replenish sodium levels.

INGREDIENTS

- 1 liter (4 cups) of water
- Juice of 2 limes
- 2 tablespoons of maple syrup
- 1/4 teaspoon (one-quarter of a teaspoon) of salt

INSTRUCTIONS

1. Combine all ingredients in a large pitcher.
2. Stir well until the salt and maple syrup are completely dissolved.
3. Chill before drinking.

Herbal Electrolyte Drink

Herbal tea adds a soothing element, while the lemon juice and honey provide essential electrolytes and energy. The salt helps maintain fluid balance.

INGREDIENTS

- 1 liter (4 cups) of water
- 1/2 (half) cup of herbal tea (like chamomile or peppermint, brewed and cooled)
- Juice of 1 lemon
- 1/4 teaspoon (one-quarter of a teaspoon) of salt
- 2 tablespoons of honey

INSTRUCTIONS

1. Brew the herbal tea and allow it to cool.
2. Mix the tea with the water, lemon juice, salt, and honey.
3. Stir well and refrigerate before drinking.

DON'T MISS YOUR BONUSES!

Make sure to get these valuable printable bonuses for FREE:

✅ Unlock **50 Extra Castor Oil Recipes** for even more health and beauty benefits

✅ Get our **Visual Castor Oil Packs Guide & 2024-2025 Calendar** to effortlessly plan your personalized castor oil treatments

✅ Discover **85 Real-life Testimonials** from people who have achieved amazing results with castor oil, and get inspired to try it yourself

✅ **Rest Easy**: explore our **Special Guide to Quality Sleep** with effective castor oil treatments

SCAN THE QR CODE BELOW
to download them:

69210528R00059